THE CERVICAL SPINE

An atlas of normal anatomy
and the morbid anatomy of
ageing and injuries

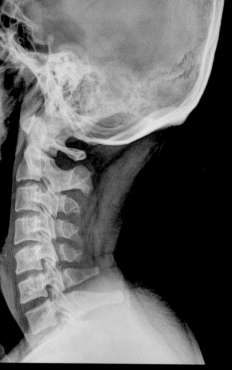

THE CERVICAL SPINE IMAGE BANK

BY JAMES TAYLOR

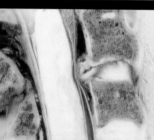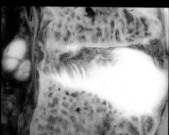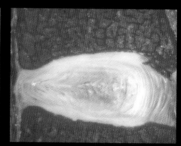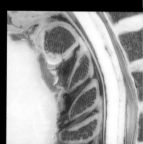

Enhance clinical understanding of cervical spine pathologies resulting from injury and ageing.

Empower students to visualize anatomical structures and develop clinical decision making skills.

Reassure and educate patients suffering from cervical spinal injury and pain.

Extracted from the text The Cervical Spine: An atlas of normal anatomy and the morbid anatomy of ageing and injuries, the entire collection of 150 unique images of normal, degenerate and injured joints, muscles and ligaments in the cervical spine is available for purchase.

KEY FEATURES:

- Image labels to highlight key features
- Systematic coverage of spinal elements, which is logical and easy to follow
- Inclusion of all anatomical features; including bone, disc, facet joints, dorsal roots

To find out more, or to buy now, visit your local Elsevier website.

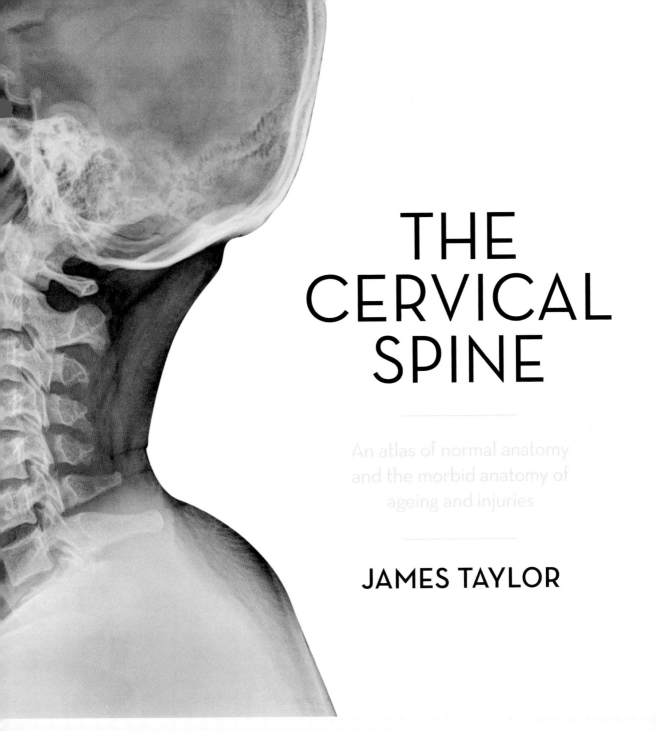

THE CERVICAL SPINE

An atlas of normal anatomy
and the morbid anatomy of
ageing and injuries

JAMES TAYLOR

ELSEVIER

ELSEVIER

Elsevier Australia. ACN 001 002 357
(a division of Reed International Books Australia Pty Ltd)
Tower 1, 475 Victoria Avenue, Chatswood, NSW 2067

Notice
This publication has been carefully reviewed and checked to ensure that the content is as accurate and current as possible at the time of publication. We would recommend, however, that the reader verifies any procedures, treatments, drug dosages or legal content described in this book. Neither the author, the contributors, nor the publisher assume any liability for injury and/or damage to persons or property arising from any error in or omission from this publication.

National Library of Australia Cataloguing-in-Publication Data

Taylor, James, 1931- author.

The cervical spine: An atlas of normal anatomy and the morbid anatomy of ageing and injuries / James Taylor.

9780729542715 (paperback).

Includes bibliographical references and index.

Spine—Abnormalities—Pictorial works.
Spine—Wounds and injuries—Pictorial works.
Spinal cord—Wounds and injuries—Pictorial works.
Whiplash injuries—Pictorial works.
Musculoskeletal diseases in old age—Pictorial works.

Senior Content Strategist: Melinda McEvoy
Content Development Specialist: Lauren Santos
Senior Project Manager: Kathryn Munro
Edited by Caroline Hunter, Burrumundi Pty Ltd
Proofread by Annabel Adair
Permissions by Sarah Thomas and Regina Remigius
Illustrations by Alan Laver (Figures 1.2, 1.3B, 1.3C, 2.6, 2.7, 2.9, 3.1A, 3.1B, 3.2, 3.6, 3.10A, 3.10B, 3.11B, 3.14B, 3.15, 3.16, 4.2, 4.3, 5.2, 9.1, 9.2, 9.3A, 9.3B, 9.4, 9.5, 9.6, 9.7)
Design by Georgette Hall
Index by Robert Swanson
Typeset by Midland Typesetters
Printed by China Translation & Printing Services Ltd

CONTENTS

FOREWORD

Professor James Taylor's book serves two main purposes: it works both as an atlas, presenting an excellent illustrated account of the development, growth, maturation and ageing of the cervical spine, while also providing text and commentary on his superb collection of slides and photographs derived from his extensive autopsy and postmortem studies. These images clearly illustrate the cervical anatomy, lesions, most vulnerable levels, and the bone and soft-tissue structures usually affected as a result of blunt trauma or motor vehicle accident (MVA) involving the neck. The images, which are unique and quite beautiful in their own right, have been widely praised and requested following his numerous conference and keynote addresses. Changes to the Coroners Act in Western Australia in 1996, bringing it into line with Acts in other states and countries, effectively restricts the potential for the removal of body parts for examination and research and it is unlikely that such extensive studies will be possible in the future.

A special focus of this text relates to whiplash-associated disorder, which so often accompanies the survivors of MVAs. Taylor makes a powerful case to assist clinicians to better understand and visualise the at-times minor bone and soft-tissue lesions that are difficult to demonstrate (even by modern scanning technologies) in whiplash patients complaining of pain and functional disturbance after what may appear to have been a relatively low-impact, rear-end vehicle collision.

Following a successful preliminary study of the autopsy records of 385 MVA victims at Royal Perth Hospital, which provided useful data confined to cervical discs and vertebral bodies (but excluding vertebral arch structures), Taylor began his major investigation of the whole cervical spines of 266 individuals as an integral part of the Royal Perth Hospital autopsy team. Detailed accounts of the subjects and sectioning/staining methodologies are included in the atlas and in the scientific papers that have been generated and presented as publications and/or at appropriate conferences. The images are clearly labelled, the anatomy/pathology is immediately recognisable to the clinical eye and they are visually dramatic. This atlas shows that many cervical spinal lesions are common to individuals who died either as a result of blunt trauma or MVA. The vexed question as to whether or not similar lesions are present in the survivors of MVA who present with whiplash symptoms is answered at least in part by Taylor's supplementary autopsy study of individuals with a history of whiplash-associated disorder who died from causes other than MVA and who showed similar lesions.

Age changes in the cervical spine are well described and demonstrated pictorially in a series of evocative images. They are seen as beginning earliest in the intervertebral discs of the subaxial spine, beginning in young adult life, which progressively show fissuring of the anulus as a natural part of the ageing process, with the nucleus becoming increasingly fibrotic and blended into the anulus until it is difficult to identify it as a discrete entity in most individuals in late middle age. Associated age changes to the vertebral bodies include uncovertebral 'joint' formation in the young, with vertebral body 'lipping' and osteophytosis following disc ageing and becoming more evident from the middle years. Osteoporosis of cervical vertebral bodies is more likely to be seen in older individuals and earlier in females than in males. The synovial joints of the upper two cervical segments and the zygapophyseal (facet) joints of the subaxial spine demonstrate age changes considerably later than do the discs. It is clinically important to differentiate age changes from those due to pathology and trauma and Taylor allows for this in the clarity with which he defines and explains 'normal' ageing changes in the region.

It has been a privilege to have been Jim's PhD student, research partner, co-author and friend since he and his family arrived in Perth in 1975. He is an extraordinary man and this book is a fitting tribute to a great teaching and research career.

Lance Twomey AO, PSBS (Malaysia), PhD BSc(Hons), BAppSc
Emeritus Professor

PREFACE

The studies reported in this atlas were undertaken in the Department of Anatomy, Physiology and Human Biology at the University of Western Australia by Professors James Taylor and Lance Twomey. The embedding of the cervical spines in low-viscosity cellulose, sectioning them on an LKB microtome and staining the sections were all done by research officer Mary Taylor with the assistance of research assistant Mary Lee (Corker). The major study of spines at Royal Perth Hospital was completed over a period of 10 years by Professor Taylor and Mary Taylor. This study was undertaken at the suggestion and with the encouragement of the late Sir George Bedbrook and at the invitation of the head of department Professor Byron Kakulas. The technical work required the essential assistance of Mary Taylor. A specially adapted precision band saw was donated to the department for the sectioning procedure by Sir George Bedbrook.

The primary purpose of the cervical spine autopsies described in this study was to assist the forensic pathologists in establishing the cause of death. All results of sectioning and photography were reported to the forensic pathologists, who included the information in their overall report to the coroner. In some cases the exact cause of death would not have been known without the information provided by sectioning the spine.

The detailed information obtained on the nature of the injuries to the head and spine helped determine the predominant direction of the forces producing the injury; for example, whether it was a blow to the face or skull vertex causing extension or compression extension, or a blow to the back of the head causing initial flexion. As noted in Professor Taylor's anatomical studies, the cervical spine is much more vulnerable to extension injury than to flexion injury as there is much less muscle protection against spinal extension and much more muscle protection against flexion of the head forwards.

Studies of cervical spine anatomy, ageing and injuries have great value for health professionals who treat spinal pain by enabling them to understand and visualise cervical spine structure and function and to see which parts of the spine are most vulnerable to pain-producing age changes or injuries. Pictorial information based on actual spinal structures is much more easily appreciated than many pages of print in a textbook and readers may well find that these images of injury and ageing illuminate the problems of the patients they see from day to day. This improved understanding of age-related pathology and injury should help health professionals in designing appropriate treatment and management regimens for their patients.

In parallel with Professor Taylor's autopsy studies, over a period of nine years he saw many patients with whiplash injuries in the pain clinic of Dr Philip Finch. This enabled Professor Taylor to compare the lesions most commonly found at autopsy with lesions that could be demonstrated in some patients.

Ethical clearance to publish the images from Professor Taylor's studies was given by the coronial ethics committee and the coroner in April 2016. Confidentiality requires that detailed information about cases that might identify the specific individual is omitted from the descriptions.

REVIEWERS

Carlos Bello
BPhty, MMuscPhty
Senior Physiotherapist, Physica Spinal &
Physiotherapy Clinic, Ringwood, Victoria;
Director, Big Hands Australia, Chirnside Park,
Victoria

Cherylea J. Browne
BMedSci (Hons), PhD
Lecturer in Human Anatomy, Western Sydney
University, New South Wales

Angie Fearon
B(AppSc)Phty, MPhty, PhD
Assistant Professor, University of Canberra,
ACT; Clinical Assistant to Professor Smith;
Visiting physiotherapist at the AIS; Director
of Hip Physio; Chair of Orthopaedic
Physiotherapy Australia (a national group of
the APA)

Toby Hall
MSc, PhD, PostGradDip Manip Ther, FACP
Adjunct Senior Teaching Fellow, Curtin
University, Perth, Western Australia

Gwendolen Jull AO
MPhty, PhD, FACP
Emeritus Professor, Physiotherapy, School
of Health and Rehabilitation Sciences,
The University of Queensland, Queensland

Kate Moss
BSc (H&SpSc) (Hons), MPhty

Sophie Paynter
BSc, BPhysio (Hons), GradCert Health Prof Ed
Senior Lecturer, Applied Anatomy
Coordinator, Physiotherapy Department,
Monash University, Victoria

Michele Sterling
BPhty, MPhty, GradDip Musc Physio, PhD, FACP
Professor, Recover Injury Research Centre,
The University of Queensland, Queensland

Benjamin K. Weeks
BPhty (Hons), BExSc, GradCert Higher Ed, PhD
Program Director, Master of Physiotherapy,
Griffith University, Queensland

Lai Kwun Yek BSc (Phty), COMT

Elsevier Australia and the author would like to acknowledge Dr Angela Fearon's valuable
contribution to the development of this publication.

ACKNOWLEDGEMENTS

My initial research on the development and growth of the human spine was extended to studies of spinal age changes during my long-term cooperation with Professor Lance Twomey. I had a long-term attachment as clinical assistant in the Sir George Bedbrook Spinal Injuries Unit at Royal Perth Rehabilitation Hospital from 1975 to 1993, which enabled me to study spinal deformities, low back pain and cervical spinal injuries.

The influence and practical support of Sir George to pursue spinal research at the University of Western Australia and in the Royal Perth Rehabilitation Hospital were an enormous encouragement and his recommendation helped us obtain research funding to enable the appointment of a research officer, Mary Taylor, and a research assistant, Mary Lee (Corker), without whom the work could not have been done. The practical work in processing the sections required the technical expertise and meticulous care provided by Mary Taylor. Over 12 years, the close teamwork made the long-term day-to-day routine of research both satisfying and effective. I thank Ken Taylor for photography of upper cervical bones.

Research funding for this study was provided by the Medical Research Fund of WA.

The facilities provided in the Department of Anatomy, Physiology and Human Biology were essential for study one. We thank Professor Byron Kakulas for the provision of two laboratories at Royal Perth Hospital, one for the band saw sectioning, the other for examination and photography of sections, and we were grateful for the ready cooperation of his staff in different stages of the autopsy examinations. As an eminent neuropathologist, Professor Kakulas provided helpful oversight and encouragement in the scientific parts of the research and his participation in the examination of injured dorsal root ganglia was essential to the success of that part of the project.

The Department of Anatomy, Physiology and Human Biology artist, Martin Thomson, drew the original professional diagrams of sections based on the rough drawings of the author. Martin's black and white drawings have been redrawn for this edition. A skilful sculptor, Hans Arkevelt, who worked in the department made beautifully accurate models of cervical vertebrae and copies were gifted to the author for use in describing vertebral anatomy.

I thank my colleague Dr Phillip Finch for his invitation to see chronic whiplash patients in his pain clinic as this gave me essential insights into the relevance of the autopsy studies to injuries in living patients. I also thank Dr Finch and his staff for their essential help and encouragement with literature searches.

Finally, I must thank Melinda McEvoy, Lauren Santos, Kathryn Munro and the staff at Elsevier Australia for their encouragement and practical help at all stages in the production and 'bringing to birth' of this work.

Professor James Taylor MB, ChB, DTM, PhD, FAFRM (Sci)
October 2016

IMAGE CREDITS

Figure 1.4, page 8: Taylor, J 2002 The pathology of whiplash: Neck sprain. *British Columbia Medical Journal*, 44, p. 253.

Figure 2.6, page 18: Taylor, J & Twomey, L 1994 Functional and applied anatomy of the cervical spine. In Grant, R (ed.), *Physical therapy of the cervical and thoracic spine*, 2nd edn, pp. 1–26. Churchill Livingstone, New York.

Figure 2.9, page 22: Taylor, J, Kakulas, B & Margolius, K 1992 Road accidents and neck injuries. *Proceedings of the Australasian Society for Human Biology*, 5, pp. 211–231.

Figure 2.13A and B, page 27: Taylor, J, Taylor, M & Twomey, L 1996 Letter to the editor. *Spine*, 21, p. 2300.

Figure 2.17, page 34: Schonstrom, N, Twomey, L & Taylor, J 1993 The lateral atlanto-axial joints and their synovial folds: An in vitro study of soft tissue injuries and fractures. *Journal of Trauma*, 35, pp. 886–892.

Figure 3.1A + C, pages 39 and 41: Taylor, J & Twomey, L 1994 Functional and applied anatomy of the cervical spine. In Grant, R (ed.), *Physical therapy of the cervical and thoracic spine*, 2nd edn, pp. 1–26. Churchill Livingstone, New York.

Figure 3.2, pages 42–43: Breathnach, A (ed.) 1958 *Frazer's anatomy of the human skeleton*. Churchill, London, p. 22.

Figure 3.4A, page 46: Taylor, JR 1974 Growth and development of the human intervertebral disc. PhD thesis, Faculty of Medicine, University of Edinburgh.

Figure 3.6, page 49: Taylor, J & Twomey, L 2000 The natural history of the lumbar spine. In *Physical therapy of the low back*, 3rd edn. Churchill Livingstone, New York.

Figure 3.10B, page 59: Adapted from Penning, L 1978 Normal movements of the cervical spine. *American Journal of Roentgenology*, 130, pp. 317–326.

Figure 3.14B, page 64: Taylor, J & Twomey, L 1994 Functional and applied anatomy of the cervical spine. In Grant, R (ed.), *Physical therapy of the cervical and thoracic spine*, 2nd edn, pp. 1–26. Churchill Livingstone, New York.

Figure 3.18, pages 68 and 69: Modified from Hoppenfeld, S 1976 *Physical examination of the spine and extremities*. Appleton Century Crofts/Prentice-Hall, New York, 1976; and Waldman, S 2015 *Physical diagnosis of pain*, 3rd edition. Elsevier, St Louis.

Figure 3.19, page 70: Adapted from Dwyer, AC, Bogduk, N & Aprill, C 1990 Cervical zygapophyseal joint pain patterns. I. A study in normal volunteers. *Spine*, 15, p. 453.

Figure 4.2, page 76: Taylor, J, Kakulas, B & Margolius, K 1992 Road accidents and neck injuries. *Proceedings of the Australasian Society for Human Biology*, 5, pp. 211–231.

Figure 4.3, page 77: Taylor, J & Twomey, L 1994 Functional and applied anatomy of the cervical spine. In Grant, R (ed.), *Physical therapy of the cervical and thoracic spine*, 2nd edn, pp. 1–26. Churchill Livingstone, New York.

Figure 4.4A, page 78: Taylor, J, Twomey, L & Levander, B 2000 Contrasts between cervical and lumbar motion segments. *Critical Reviews in Physical and Rehabilitation Medicine*, 12, pp. 345–371.

Figure 5.1A, page 96: Taylor, JR & Taylor, M 1996 Cervical spine injuries: An autopsy study of 109 blunt injuries. *Journal of Musculoskeletal Pain*, 4, pp. 61–79.

Figure 5.2, page 99: Taylor, JR 1993 Neck sprain. *Australian Family Physician*, 22, pp. 1623–1629.

Figure 5.4B, page 103: Taylor, JR & Taylor, M 1996 Cervical spine injuries: An autopsy study of 109 blunt injuries. *Journal of Musculoskeletal Pain*, 4, pp. 61–79.

Figure 5.6A, page 106: Taylor, JR & Taylor, M 1996 Cervical spine injuries: An autopsy study of 109 blunt injuries. *Journal of Musculoskeletal Pain*, 4, pp. 61–79.

Figure 5.8, page 109: Taylor, J & Kakulas, B 1991 Neck injuries. *The Lancet*, 338, p. 1343.

Figure 5.13A, page 118: Finch, P & Taylor, J 1996 Functional anatomy of the spine. In Waldeman, S & Winnie, A (eds), *Interventional pain management*. Saunders, Philadelphia.

Figure 6.4A, page 128: Taylor, J, Twomey, L & Kakulas, B 1998 Dorsal root ganglion injuries in 109 blunt trauma fatalities. *Injury*, 29, pp. 335–339.

Figure 7.3A, page 140: Taylor, J & Taylor, M 1996 Cervical spinal injuries: An autopsy study of 109 blunt injuries. *Journal of Musculoskeletal Pain*, 4, pp. 61–77.

Figure 7.5B, page 145: Finch, P & Taylor, J 1996 Functional anatomy of the spine. In Waldeman, S & Winnie, A (eds), *Interventional pain management*. Saunders, Philadelphia.

Figure 8.13B, page 169: Cheong, WY & Tan, KP 1991 Air in the cervical annulus: The lucent cleft sign. *Singapore Medical Journal*, 32, pp. 255–257.

FIGURE REFERENCE GUIDE

This atlas presents pictures of normal, degenerate and injured joints, muscles and ligaments in the cervical spine, garnered from a study of 266 autopsies covering a period of almost 10 years. It contains more than 150 pictures and diagrams crammed with information.

AIMS OF THE ATLAS

The aims of the atlas are to:
- illustrate the functional anatomy of normal, young cervical spines based on examination of serial sagittal and coronal sections
- describe and illustrate age changes in the cervical spine, showing how degenerative changes alter function and may cause pain and disability
- describe and portray the nature, frequency and distribution of cervical spine injuries due to blunt trauma, based on autopsy examinations of 162 injured cervical spines from blunt trauma deaths, compared with 104 autopsy examinations with no history of acute blunt trauma (the injury study is mainly concerned with injuries in well-aligned spines, which account for about half of the 162 cases)
- compare the pathology of common lesions seen in well-aligned spines with lesions that can be demonstrated in whiplash patients
- examine the spines of a smaller subgroup of subjects with a history of whiplash injury who died of other causes for 'whiplash lesions'
- seek to answer the question often posed, 'Does chronic whiplash-associated disorder (WAD) have lesions that help explain the pain?'
- demonstrate the 'weaker areas' of the cervical spine based on the high frequency of lesions at particular sites
- show clinicians where to look for likely whiplash injury lesions, based on data on the frequency and situation of blunt trauma lesions.

In particular, this study focuses on a comparison of autopsy lesions in well-aligned spines with whiplash lesions in living patients. Whiplash lesions in living patients may be difficult or sometimes impossible to demonstrate, but portrayal of these lesser injuries found consistently at autopsy can help clinicians to forecast where whiplash lesions are most likely to occur. Bogduk and others (Bogduk, 2006; Curatolo, Bogduk, Ivancic et al., 2011) claim that whiplash patients must have physical lesions to account for their ongoing, well-identified, localised pain, although they have been unable to demonstrate those lesions.

THE UNIQUE STRUCTURE OF THE CERVICAL SPINE

The cervical spine is unique in its structure and function for several reasons:

1. *It is by far the most slender and mobile region of the human spine, especially in its range of axial rotation.* It can move the 4-kilogram head to direct the gaze to the right, left, up or down. This mobility is especially due to the wide range of movement (ROM) in the synovial joints of the upper two cervical segments but is also due to the wider ROM per segment in the subaxial segments compared to the thoracic and lumbar segments.

2. *The orientation of the cervical zygapophyseal facets at 45° to the long axis of the spine differs from facet orientation in the thoracic and lumbar spine.* From C2–3 to C4–5 the 45° facets determine the nature of the subaxial movements. The centres of motion for these segments are well below the discs, as sagittal plane rotation is coupled with sagittal plane translation or forward/backward slide. This translation results in high shearing strains in the cervical intervertebral discs.

3. *The upward growth of uncinate processes at the lateral margins of vertebral bodies in childhood is unique to the cervical spine.* Their growth narrows the lateral intervertebral spaces and results in the formation of uncovertebral clefts at the lateral margins of the cervical discs by puberty.

4. *The passage of large vertebral arteries, upwards through the transverse foramina (foramina transversaria) of all vertebrae from C6 to C1, is unique to the cervical spine.* The arteries pass through the foramen magnum into the cranial cavity to supply the hindbrain.

5. *There is a uniquely marked contrast between the small anterior muscles of the cervical spine and the large mass of its posterior muscles.*

6. *The cervical discs are uniquely fissured in early adult life by the medial spread of fissures from the uncovertebral clefts.* The same shearing forces that form uncovertebral clefts extend fissures medially through the central and posterior parts of the cervical discs. By the age of 40–45 years, the anterior annulus and the two longitudinal ligaments are the only intact structures joining adjacent vertebral bodies together. Early disc fissuring and the stresses of the wide range of cervical mobility contribute to disc degeneration in middle and later adult life. The most mobile discs at C5–6 and C6–7 frequently show the formation of marginal osteophytes. These may impinge on spinal nerves, vertebral arteries and the spinal cord.

7. *The cervical spine is uniquely vulnerable to extension (whiplash) trauma.* The very slender structure of the cervical spine which helps give it its wide range of mobility also makes it vulnerable to trauma. It is especially vulnerable to extension trauma, as its flexor muscles are so much smaller than its extensors. The deep flexors—the thin, strap-like anterior longus colli muscles—are much weaker than the large mass of the posterior muscles, even when supported by the lateral sternocleidomastoid muscles. Blunt trauma to the cervical spine occurs most often in motor vehicle accidents, classically in rear-end collisions, but also in falls in the elderly with frontal blows to the head.

THE AIMS OF THE AUTOPSY STUDIES

In this atlas we present pictorial information of normal anatomy, age changes in anatomy and the morbid anatomy of injuries in the upper cervical region and the subaxial region of the cervical spine from observations and photography in many autopsies and a few dissecting room cadavers. We also compare the injuries in well-aligned spines with whiplash injury lesions in living patients. Studies of the sites and frequency of lesions due to blunt trauma reveal which parts of the spine are most vulnerable to injury and throw light on the soft-tissue injuries and minor fractures most likely to occur in moderate to severe whiplash injuries, where x-rays are unable to reveal the injury.

Full descriptions of blunt trauma lesions in discs, facet joints, dorsal root ganglia and other structures are provided in Chapters 5 to 8, with an emphasis on injuries likely to occur in whiplash.

Dorsal root ganglion injuries were commonly found and are also described in detail elsewhere (see Taylor, Twomey & Kakulas, 1998).

The first part of this study was conducted in the Department of Anatomy and Human Biology at the University of Western Australia (UWA). The success of this study led to the author being invited by Professor Byron Kakulas, the Head of Neuropathology, to perform spinal autopsies in the Department of Pathology at Royal Perth Hospital (RPH). It was a great privilege to assist the forensic pathologists who had the responsibility of determining the cause of death in coroners' cases. At the same time, we were able to research the nature of cervical spinal injuries in deaths from blunt trauma.

In a preliminary study of the extensive autopsy records from 385 road accident deaths at RPH, we found that half of all the spinal injuries recorded were in the cervical spine, where injuries to the intervertebral discs at the disc–vertebral body junction were much more common than fractures to vertebral bodies. However, the RPH reports of spinal autopsies were limited to studies of x-rays and midline sections after laminectomy to extract the spinal cord. These limited procedures would have missed most facet joint injuries.

We report detailed observations of serial sections of whole cervical spines at RPH in the period from 1989 to June 1996 when a new coronial Act restricted the possibility of examining cervical spines removed from cadavers. The current coronial Act takes account of the rights of the next of kin of the deceased to object to autopsy examination and in particular to object to the removal of body parts for special examination. This probably makes our extensive study, performed under the previous Act, unique in modern times.

Study methodology

In total in this study, cervical spines from 266 individuals were examined by two different methods.

The first part of the study, performed in the Department of Anatomy and Human Biology at UWA, examined 32 cervical spines ranging from 14 to 80 years of age; 16 were from deaths due to blunt trauma and 16 had no history of trauma (Taylor & Twomey, 1993). Figure 1.1 shows how these spines were sectioned. The spines were fixed in formalin, then dehydrated and embedded in low-viscosity nitrocellulose in a process that took about 3 months for the larger blocks of tissue. The embedded blocks were then sectioned at 100 microns thickness on an LKB microtome. The sections were stained by haematoxylin and counterstained by light green and mounted on glass slides for microscopy and photography. This method is described in detail in Giles and Taylor (1983) and Taylor (1974). Each block was sectioned in the sagittal plane up to the midline, then turned 90° to section the remainder in the coronal plane. Sagittal plane sections demonstrate the facet joints well and the coronal sections are best suited to show the uncus, uncovertebral clefts and age-related fissures.

The second, much larger, part of the study conducted in the Department of Pathology at RPH examined 234 cervical spines of all ages from early childhood up to individuals over 80 years of age; 88 spines had no history of injury and 146 were from blunt trauma deaths, including 95 deaths in road accidents and 51 deaths due to falls or blows to the head. The 88 spines with no history or evidence of blunt trauma served as 'controls' for the studies of blunt trauma injuries. The majority of cervical spines autopsied were from relatively young subjects: two-thirds were in the age range 10 to 49 years. From age 50 to 79 years there was a progressive decrease in numbers with advancing age, but there was an increase in numbers in the 80–89 age group. Many of the elderly subjects died from falls or blows to the head. Head injuries were the most common cause of death, but severe torso injuries without external evidence of head impact were also common.

For these cases, examined at the request of the forensic pathologists, the whole cervical spine was expertly removed from the cadaver by a laboratory technician and fixed by immersion in formalin for 7 to 10 days. We then embedded the spine, correctly oriented, in 6.5% warm gelatin solution in a suitable container (Figure 1.2) and deep froze it on dry ice at –70° C for 24–48 hours. The gelatin-enclosed block was sagittally sectioned in 2.5 mm thick serial slices on a specially adapted band saw with a precision-adjustable guide and a fine-toothed blade (Figure 1.5). The enclosure in gelatin before freezing allowed sectioning without damage to the surface of the spinal tissues as the blade passed smoothly from the frozen gelatin into the frozen spinal tissues. We wore two pairs of rubber gloves when handling the block to avoid cold burns.

Each slice was carefully washed and cleared of saw-cut debris and placed underwater in a large Petri dish to be photographed using a Pentax camera with a macro lens. Each slice was examined under an M3 Leitz dissecting microscope at low magnification and pictures were taken of injuries or other structures of interest. Photography underwater was necessary to avoid distortion by reflection of light from the surface of the section. We calculated that about 0.6 mm of tissue was lost or worn away by the saw blade between successive sections and there were usually 14 to 16 sections per spine. Sections were

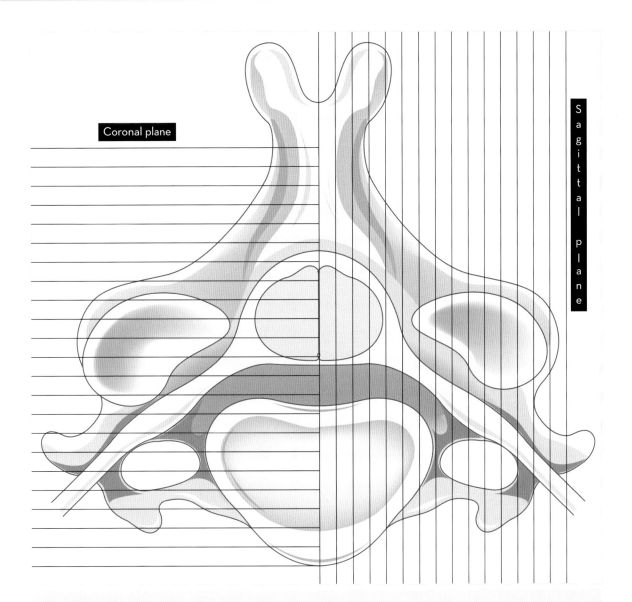

FIGURE 1.1
Study methodology.

Method of sectioning the first group of 32 spines. Each block was sectioned first in the sagittal plane to the midline, then turned 90° to section the remaining half in the coronal plane.

stored between numbered sheets of paper in 70% alcohol until the whole forensic examination of the case was complete. A written report on the nature and extent of injuries or other findings of interest was prepared for the forensic pathologist. This was included in the pathologist's report to the coroner to establish the cause and mechanism of death.

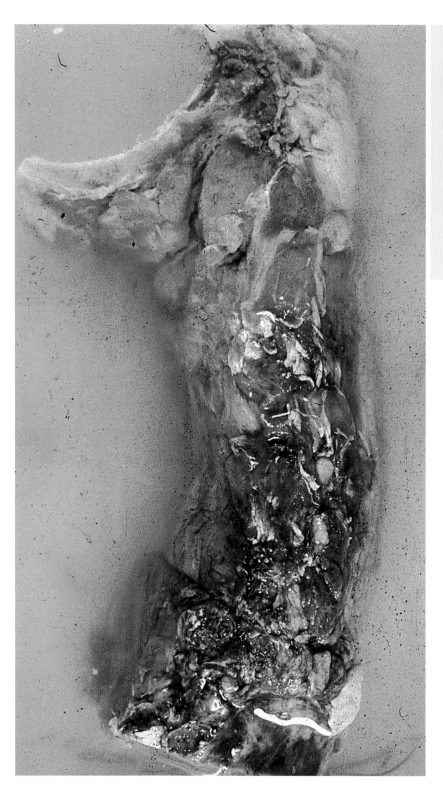

**FIGURE 1.2
Sample
preparation.**

The whole cervical
spine, including
part of the base
of the skull, was
fixed in formalin,
then embedded in
gelatin. The spine
is viewed from the
side, suitably oriented
for sectioning in the
sagittal plane.

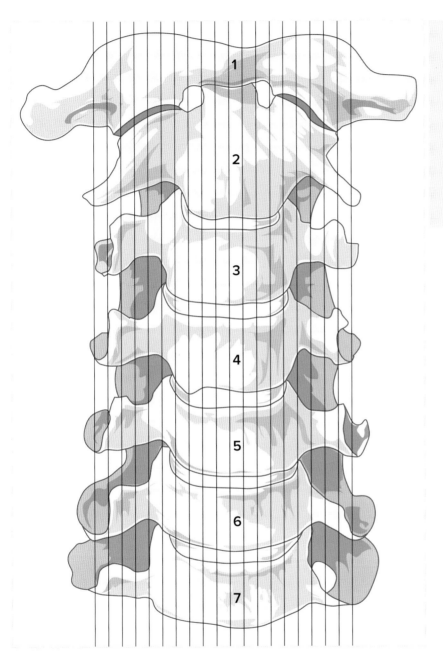

FIGURE 1.3
Sectioning diagram.

The plane of sectioning shown on a diagram of an anterior view of the cervical spine. In study 2, all spines were sectioned in the sagittal plane unless stated otherwise.

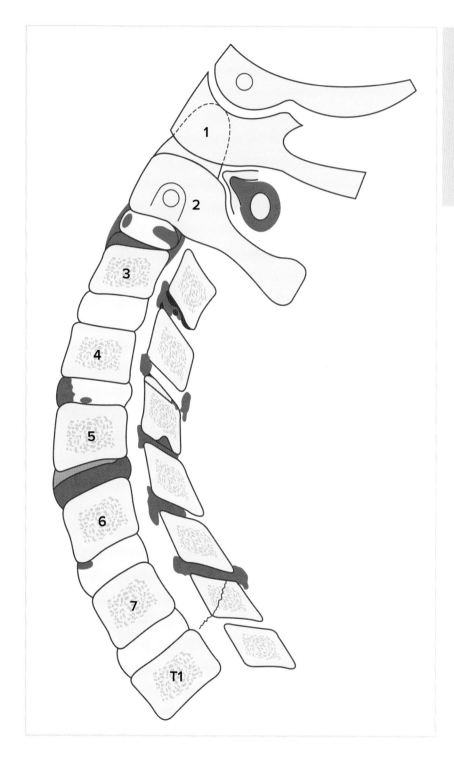

FIGURE 1.4

A record of injuries diagram.

Standard diagrams were used to record the nature and position of all the injuries observed on right and left (Taylor, 2002).

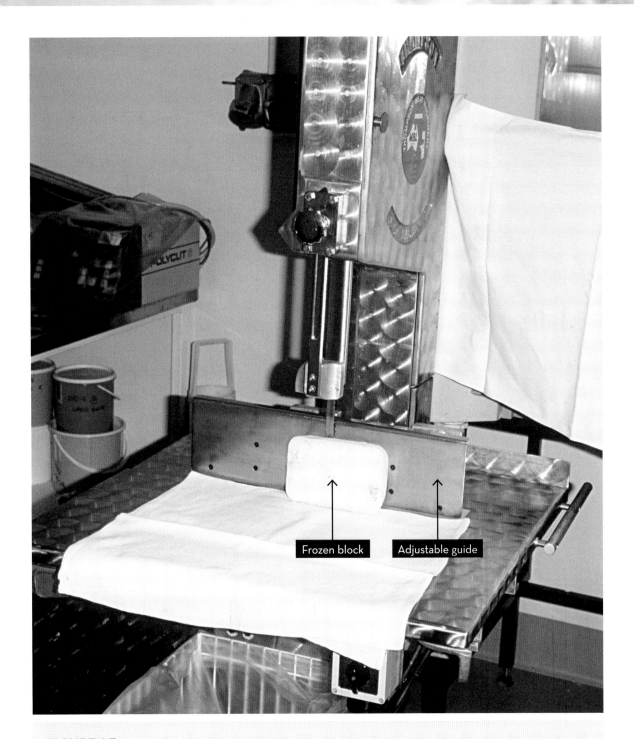

Frozen block   Adjustable guide

FIGURE 1.5
Saw table.

The saw table with the large adjustable, precision guide (to regulate section thickness); a frozen block lies on the table, ready to be sectioned.

CHAPTER 2

ANATOMY AND INJURIES IN UPPER CERVICAL VERTEBRAE AND JOINTS

ANATOMY OF UPPER CERVICAL VERTEBRAE AND JOINTS

The cervical spine has two quite distinct regions: from C2–3 down to the sacrum all intervertebral joints include an intervertebral disc and two facet joints. By contrast, the bones and synovial joints of the upper two segments are so different from those of the subaxial spine that it is best to deal with them separately. The atlas (C1) and the axis (C2) are joined to each other and to the skull base only by synovial joints supported by strong ligaments. This makes their joints much more mobile than the disc plus two facet joints at each subaxial segment. The atlanto-occipital (C0–1) and atlanto-axial (C1–2) synovial joints together give about 50% of the total cervical ranges of movement.

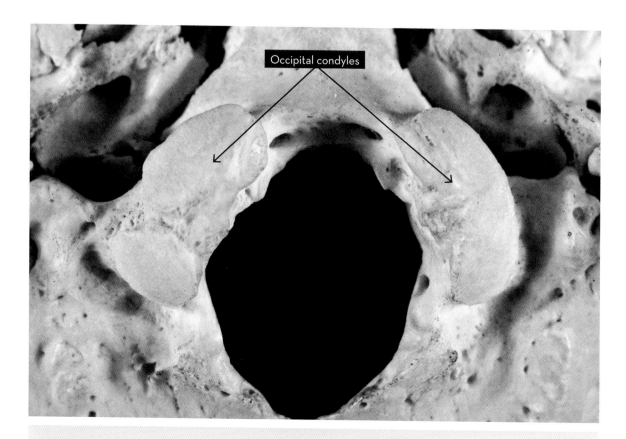

FIGURE 2.1

The occipital condyles for the atlanto-occipital (C0–1) joints.

The anterior part of the foramen magnum is flanked by the convex occipital condyles, which articulate with the concave upper facets on the lateral masses of C1. (Normally each condyle has a single oval articular surface. In this elderly adult the joint surface of the left condyle is in two parts.)

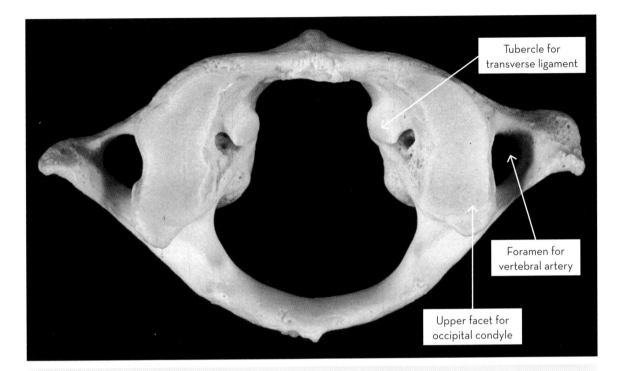

Tubercle for
transverse ligament

Foramen for
vertebral artery

Upper facet for
occipital condyle

FIGURE 2.2
The atlas (C1) viewed from above.

Two lateral masses are joined by a short anterior arch and a long posterior arch. C1 has no centrum and therefore no vertebral body. Its spinal canal is very large. The anterior part of this space is for the dens of the axis (C2), which articulates with the anterior arch of C1. The dens is held in place by a strong transverse ligament attached to the tubercles medial to the upper facets. The wider posterior part of the spinal canal contains the dural sac with its contents, the spinal cord bathed in cerebrospinal fluid. The transverse processes of C1 are long with transverse foramina to transmit the vertebral arteries. The vertebral arteries then pass around behind the lateral masses of C1, in grooves on its posterior arch. The paired vertebral arteries pass up through the foramen magnum to anastomose with the internal carotid arteries in the circle of Willis. They supply the hindbrain and the cervical spinal cord.

The concave oval facets on the upper surfaces of the lateral masses of C1 articulate with the convex facets on the occipital condyles. These joints with their supporting muscles balance and move the 4-kilogram head. The atlas facets slope downwards and medially so that an axial force from a blow to the skull vertex would tend to force the two lateral masses apart, as in a Jefferson fracture of the anterior and posterior arches. (In this image the small holes next to the tubercles for the transverse ligaments are artefacts made when articulating the skeleton.)

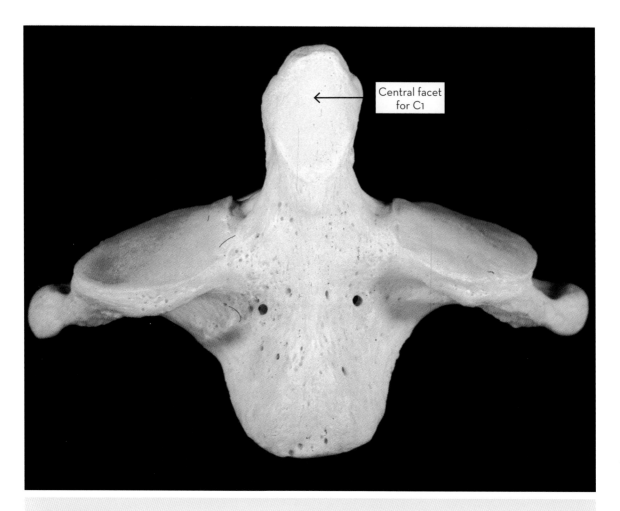

Central facet
for C1

FIGURE 2.3A

The axis (C2) seen from in front.

The dens (or odontoid process) surmounts the C2 vertebral body. The facets on the lateral masses slope downwards and laterally; they are convex in the sagittal plane. The dens is the pivot around which the head can be turned to the left or the right.

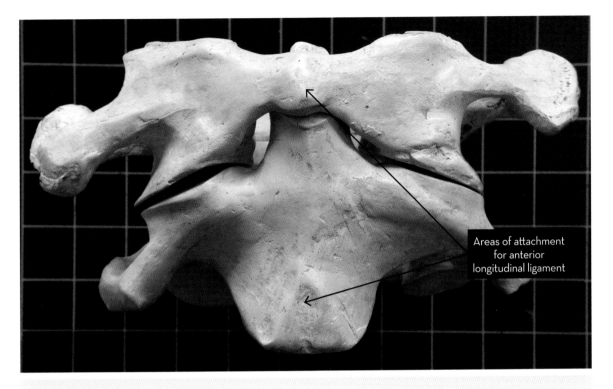

Areas of attachment
for anterior
longitudinal ligament

FIGURE 2.3B

C1 and C2 viewed from the front.

The raised triangular area on the anterior surface of the body of C2 and the small tubercle at the centre of the anterior arch of C1 mark the upper areas of attachment of the strong anterior longitudinal ligament which ascends on the anterior surface of the spine to its uppermost attachment on the tubercle of C1.

The lateral atlanto-axial (C1–2) joint facets slope downwards and laterally; they are flat in the coronal plane but biconvex in the sagittal plane (Figures 2.8 and 2.9). This biconvexity leaves gaps at the front and back which are filled in life by vascular fat-filled synovial folds. The incongruous C1–2 lateral joints differ significantly in shape from the congruous lateral atlanto-occipital (Co–1) joints, where the convex occipital condyles on the skull base fit neatly into the concave facets on the lateral masses of C1 (Figure 2.8A).

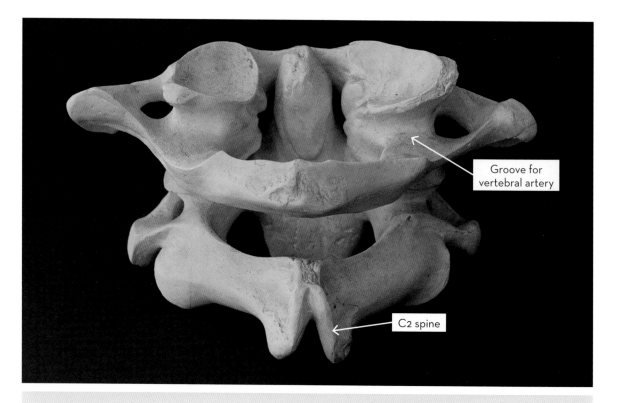

Groove for
vertebral artery

C2 spine

FIGURE 2.4
A view of C1 and C2 articulated, seen from behind and slightly above.

The concave upper facets on C1 articulate with the occipital condyles and the dens articulates with the anterior arch of C1. The groove for the vertebral artery runs medially from the transverse foramen on the posterior arch of C1. The posterior arch of C1 is not prominent but its upper surface is grooved by the vertebral arteries. By contrast, C2 has a large, strong spinous process shaped like an inverted V. It is an important suboccipital landmark; many muscles converge to attach to it, including the strong extensor semispinalis cervicis from below, the small inferior oblique muscles from the sides and the rectus capitis posterior major from above.

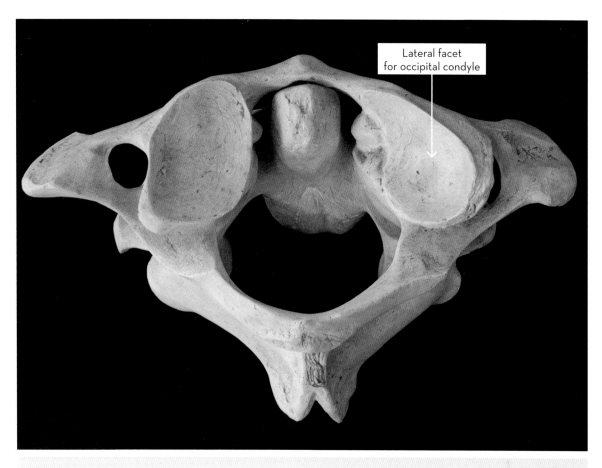

Lateral facet
for occipital condyle

FIGURE 2.5
C1 and C2 articulated, viewed from above.

The anterior spinal canal is occupied by the dens, and the posterior part of the canal would contain the dural sac with the spinal cord. The strong spine of C2 projects back beyond the posterior arch of C1.

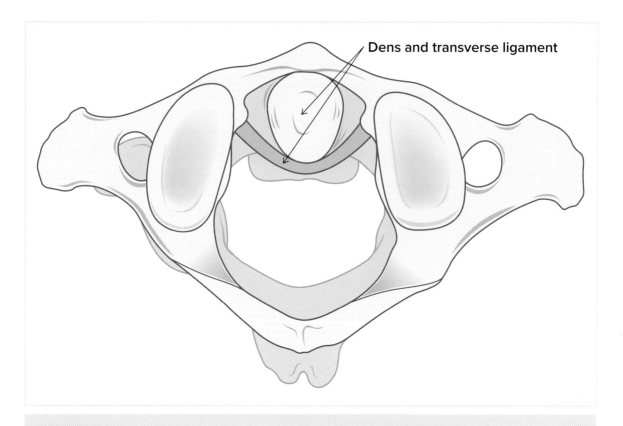

Dens and transverse ligament

FIGURE 2.6

A diagram of C1 and C2 articulated, viewed from above.

The transverse ligament anchors the dens in place, preventing its backwards dislocation, but it allows free axial rotation around the dens as its fulcrum. Synovial cavities line both the front and the back of the dens, lubricating its movement on the anterior arch of the atlas within the encircling transverse ligament. The transverse ligament intersects with smaller vertical collagen fibres forming a 'cruciate' ligament, but the transverse ligament is the strongest and most important element. Its integrity is essential for stability in rotation. The strong transverse and alar ligaments are essential to the stability of the upper cervical spine.

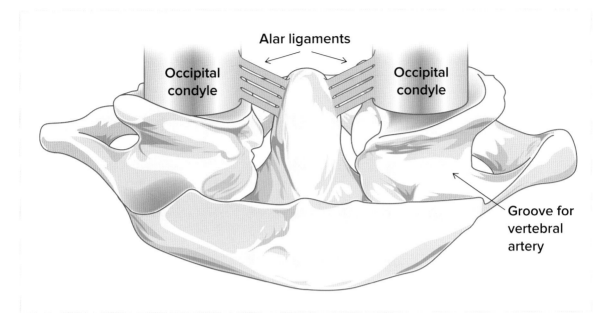

FIGURE 2.7

A view of the dens from behind, where it articulates with the anterior arch of C1 and with the transverse ligament.

On each side of the dens is a diagrammatic representation of the occipital condyles. The alar ligaments attach the upper lateral aspects of the dens to each occipital condyle. These strong ligaments pass upwards and laterally like 'wings'. Their old name 'check ligaments' indicates their function of allowing axial rotation but 'checking it' at end-range.

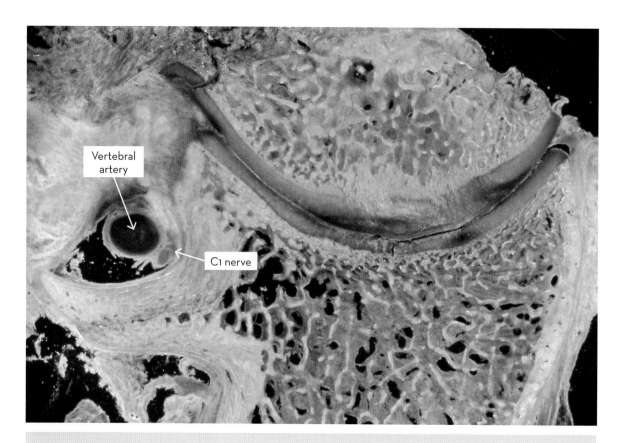

FIGURE 2.8A

A sagittal section of the atlanto-occipital (C0–1) joint.

A 100-micron unstained sagittal section of the lateral C0–1 joint was photographed with dark ground illumination. This normal joint is from a 16-year-old youth. The congruous joint surfaces of the occipital condyle and the lateral mass of C1 look well suited to flexion and extension in the sagittal plane. The vertebral artery is traversing the groove on the posterior arch of C1 with the small first cervical nerve under it. The C1 nerve supplies the small suboccipital muscles, inferior oblique, superior oblique and rectus capitis posterior major and minor.

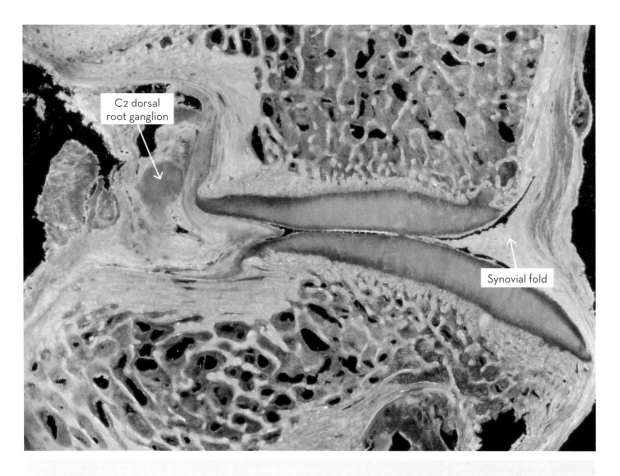

FIGURE 2.8B
A sagittal section of the atlanto-axial (C1–2) joint from a 16-year-old youth.

The biconvex surfaces are incongruous. Triangular vascular synovial folds occupy the spaces in front and back of the biconvex C1–2 joints. The C2 dorsal root ganglion lies in vascular areolar tissue directly behind the C1–2 joint. The range of sagittal plane movement is almost as wide at C1–2 as at C0–1 but the smooth gliding movements of C0–1 contrast with the rolling movements at C1–2.

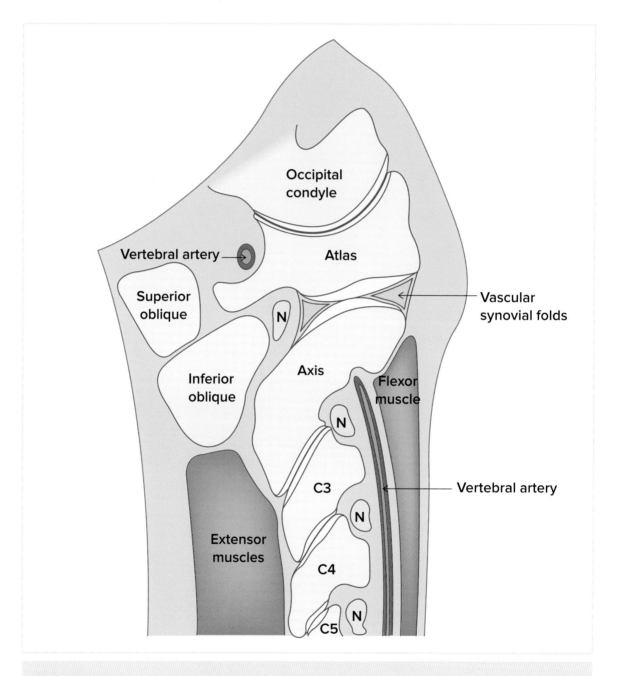

FIGURE 2.9

A diagram based on a sagittal section of the upper cervical spine.

The diagram shows the more anterior position of Co–1 and C1–2 compared to the zygapophyseal facet joints. Note the contrast between the large posterior extensor muscles and the small anterior flexor muscle.

N = spinal nerve.

TABLE 2.1	Ranges of movement at C0–1 and C1–2	
	C0–1	**C1–2**
Flexion	3.5°	11.5°
Extension	21.0°	10.9°
Side-bending (one side)	10.9°	6.7°
Axial rotation (one side)	6.7°	38.9°

Source: Panjabi, M, Dvorak, J, Duranceau, J et al. 1988 Three-dimensional movement of the upper cervical spine. *Spine*, 13, pp. 726–727.

The sum of sagittal plane flexion extension for C0–1 is 24.5° and for C1–2 it is 22.4°. Note the very large range of axial rotation at C1–2, which is recorded by other authors as 40° in each direction (Penning, 1968; Penning, 1978).

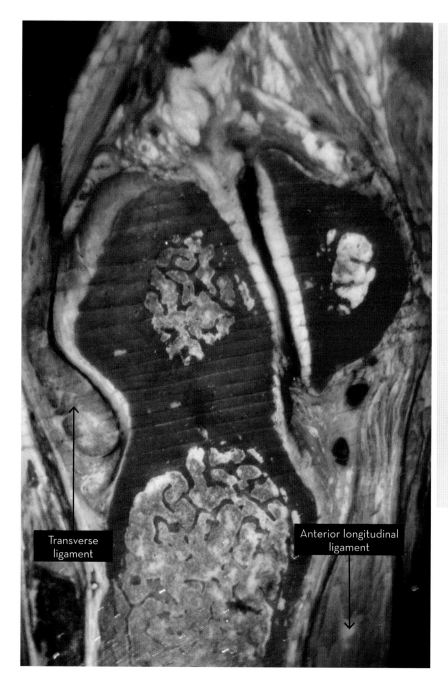

Transverse ligament

Anterior longitudinal ligament

FIGURE 2.10
The midline atlanto-axial joints.

An Alizarin-stained section shows the joint between the dens and the anterior arch of the atlas, and the joint between the dens and the transverse ligament. The dens is held in place by the transverse ligament, which grooves the posterior surface of the dens (there is artefact damage to the ligament). These joints allow a wide range of axial rotation to the right and left around the fulcrum of the dens. The anterior longitudinal ligament passes up in front of the C2 vertebral body to attach to the anterior arch of the atlas.

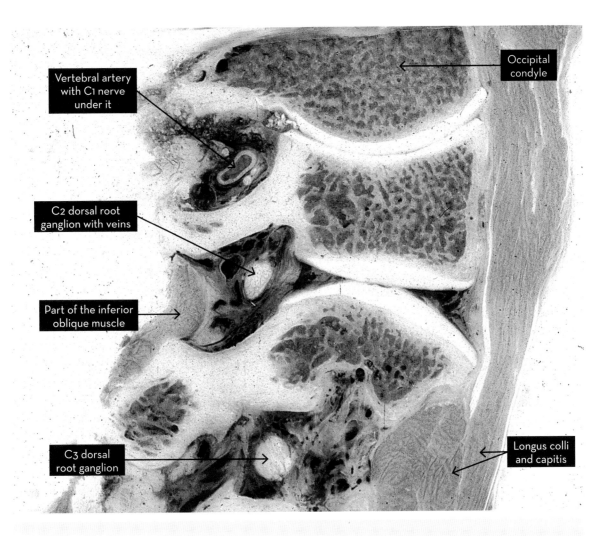

FIGURE 2.11

A thick unstained sagittal section through the lateral C0–1 and C1–2 joints.

The C0–1 and C1–2 joints lie directly above the vertebral bodies and discs; they are supplied by the ventral rami of C1 and C2. The zygapophyseal facets are on a more posterior plane and are supplied segmentally by medial branches of dorsal rami. The anterior alignment of C1 and C2 leaves a suboccipital space behind C1 and C2, below the occipital bone and above the prominent C2–3 facets. This space contains the vertebral artery on the posterior arch of C1, with the small C1 nerve between the artery and the arch. Behind C1–2 the dorsal root ganglion of C2 is surrounded by a venous plexus. The space is partly 'enclosed' by the inferior oblique muscle and its strong capsular covering. The suboccipital muscles are innervated by C1 and C2 dorsal rami. The longus colli and capitis are closely applied to the anterior surfaces of C1 and C2 and are supplied by upper cervical ventral rami.

The venous plexus around the C2 dorsal root ganglion is formed by the confluence of the two valveless longitudinal venous sinuses from the anterior epidural space with vertebral veins and deep cervical veins. These veins are said to be subject to arteriolar pressures and may become congested (Parke, 1978; Jansen et al., 1989).

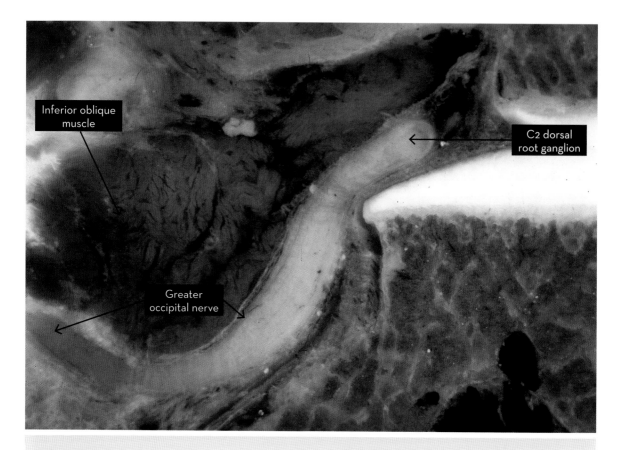

FIGURE 2.12

The greater occipital nerve.

The greater occipital nerve originates behind the C1–2 lateral joint. It is one of the largest cutaneous nerves in the body. It is the medial branch of the dorsal ramus of C2. To reach the occipital skin the nerve arches downwards below the inferior oblique muscle and then upwards through the semispinalis and the tendinous part of the trapezius. This nerve is vulnerable to irritation by venous engorgement at its origin or by tightness in the semispinalis or trapezius, causing occipital neuritis.

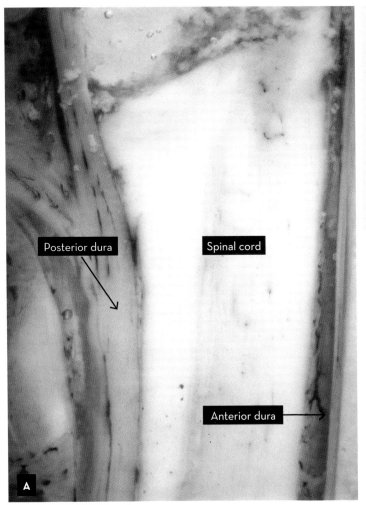

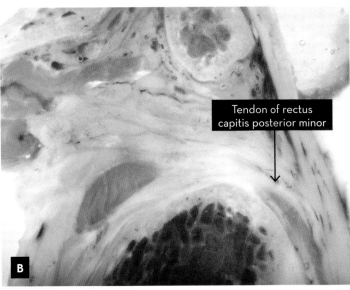

FIGURE 2.13A AND B
The upper cervical dura mater at the C1–2 level.

The upper posterior dura is consistently several times thicker than the anterior dura **(A)**. This is because part of the rectus capitis posterior minor inserts into the posterior dura **(B)**. Muscle contraction prevents buckling of the dura onto the cord during neck extension.

UPPER CERVICAL INJURIES: FRACTURES

Upper cervical fractures or dislocations were common in severe blunt trauma with head injuries, causing fatal, high spinal cord injury (SCI). These atlanto-occipital or atlanto-axial dislocations with fatal spinal cord injury are the province of pathologists rather than clinicians.

Schonstrom, Twomey and Taylor (1993) have published descriptions of injuries to atlanto-axial joints. The dens fracture was often found in old subjects with a stiff lower cervical spine. Lower cervical stiffness made the upper levels more vulnerable to injury from simple falls with head impact and forced extension. Jain (2015) records a marked recent increase in the prevalence of cord injury in the elderly due to falls.

This account focuses on injuries in well-aligned spines and an example of a small compression fracture of bony trabeculae involving the lateral C1–2 joint is shown (Figure 2.14), along with two examples of upper cervical fractures: a dens fracture (Figure 2.15A) and a hangman fracture (Figure 2.15B) .

Small trabecular compression fractures without fracture dislocation were relatively common in the upper cervical region involving the occipital condyles and the lateral masses of the atlas and the axis vertebrae.

The dens fracture (Figure 2.15A) is accompanied by a fatal upper spinal cord injury and the hangman fracture (Figure 2.15B) shows posterior displacement of the vertebral arch and anterior herniation of part of the C2–3 disc. Both dens and hangman fractures can occur without cord injury and are important clinically. Dens fracture were the most common upper cervical fractures in this study.

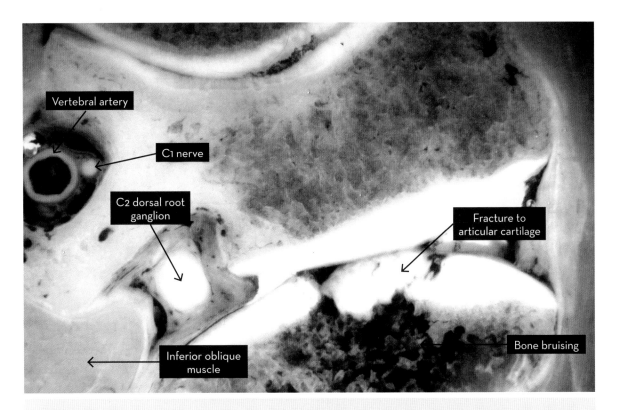

FIGURE 2.14

A compression injury to the lower articular cartilage and subchondral bone of C1–2 with multiple trabecular fractures (bone bruising) in the lateral mass of C2.

The C2 dorsal root ganglion lies immediately behind the C1–2 joint between the joint and the inferior oblique muscle. The vertebral artery lies on the posterior arch of C1 with the small first cervical nerve between the artery and the bone.

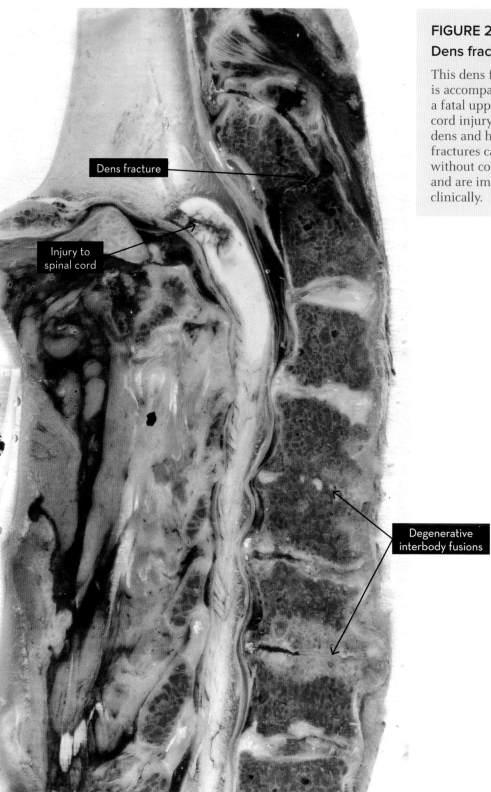

Dens fracture

Injury to
spinal cord

Degenerative
interbody fusions

FIGURE 2.15A
Dens fracture.

This dens fracture
is accompanied by
a fatal upper spinal
cord injury but both
dens and hangman
fractures can occur
without cord injury
and are important
clinically.

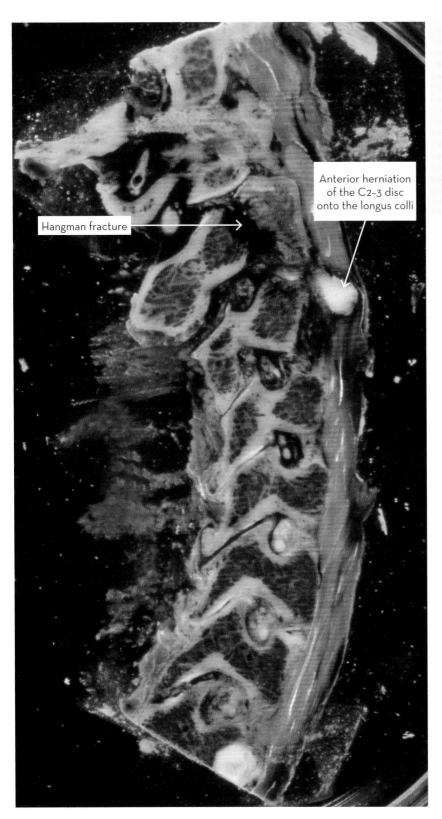

Hangman fracture

Anterior herniation of the C2-3 disc onto the longus colli

FIGURE 2.15B
Hangman fracture.

The hangman fracture is a bilateral fracture of the vertebral arch. The injury on one side is shown; it was mirrored by a similar fracture on the other side.

UPPER CERVICAL INJURIES: SOFT-TISSUE INJURIES

The exceedingly common injury of posterior synovial fold (meniscal) bruising was seen in subjects with head extension trauma from head impacts. An injury to the veins of the suboccipital venous plexus often accompanied this. The majority of head injury deaths showed bruising of the posterior meniscus or, less often, of both menisci in the C1–2 lateral joints. Posterior bruising often extended backwards around the C2 dorsal root ganglion and nerve, forming a large haematoma which might track along the course of the greater occipital nerve. These menisci move in and out of the joint during normal movements in life but in the few milliseconds of a car accident they are caught, compressed and bruised.

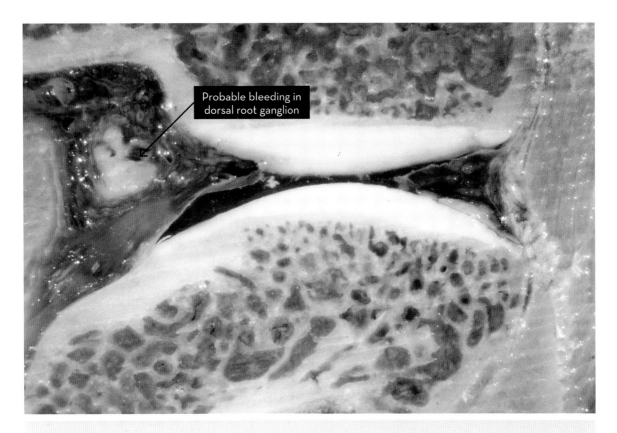

Probable bleeding in
dorsal root ganglion

FIGURE 2.16
A sagittal section showing bruising of both the posterior and the anterior synovial folds.

There appears to be bleeding into the C2 dorsal root ganglion with two small areas of
haemorrhage.

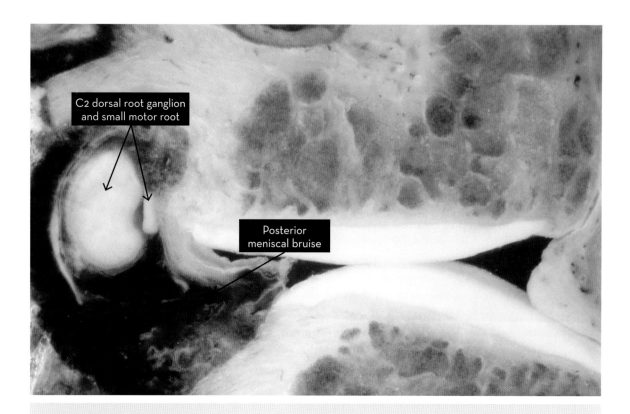

FIGURE 2.17A
A sagittal section of C1–2 showing bleeding into the posterior synovial fold (meniscus).

This was by far the most common upper cervical injury in this study. The rapid extension movement nips and bruises the vascular fold. The bleeding may extend backwards into the areolar tissue behind the joint surrounding the dorsal root ganglion. The contrast in size between the large ganglion and the small motor root is clearly seen.

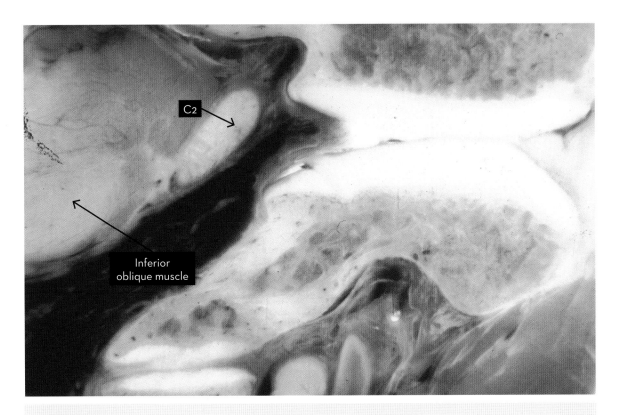

FIGURE 2.17B
A sagittal section showing a haematoma behind the C1–2 lateral joint.

The large haematoma extends from the posterior part of the joint along the course of the greater occipital nerve under the inferior oblique muscle. Such an injury may involve the venous plexus around the nerve and in a survivor it would be likely to cause an occipital headache.

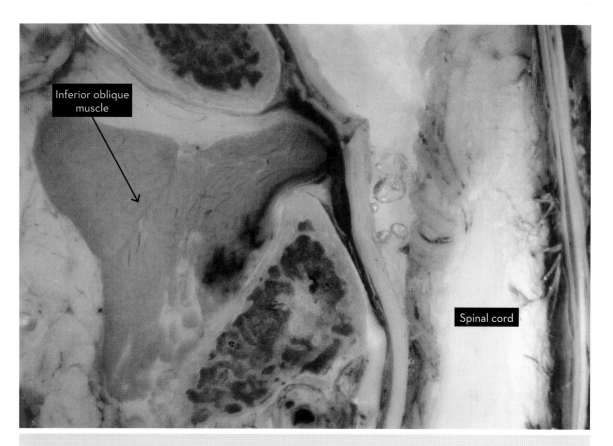

Inferior oblique muscle

Spinal cord

FIGURE 2.18

A sagittal section showing a less common injury due to the nipping of the inferior oblique muscle between the posterior arches of C1 and C2 in an extension injury.

These injuries occur during the very rapid movements in motor vehicle accidents.

RELATIONSHIP OF UPPER CERVICAL INJURIES TO HEAD INJURIES

In the autopsy studies, upper cervical injuries were most often secondary to head injuries. The injuries at Co–1 and C1–2 were less common in torso injuries where there was no external evidence of head impact. This was especially noted in severe upper cervical fractures or dislocations. Soft-tissue injuries to the C1–2 synovial folds were also more common in deaths from head injuries but they were also common in torso injuries without evidence of head impact.

A careful examination of the frequency of subaxial cervical injuries to discs, facets and other cervical tissues comparing head injuries to torso injuries found closely comparable frequency and distribution of injuries in the two groups. Lesions in discs and facets were very similar in position and frequency when comparing cases of head injuries with cases of torso injuries where there was no evidence of head impact.

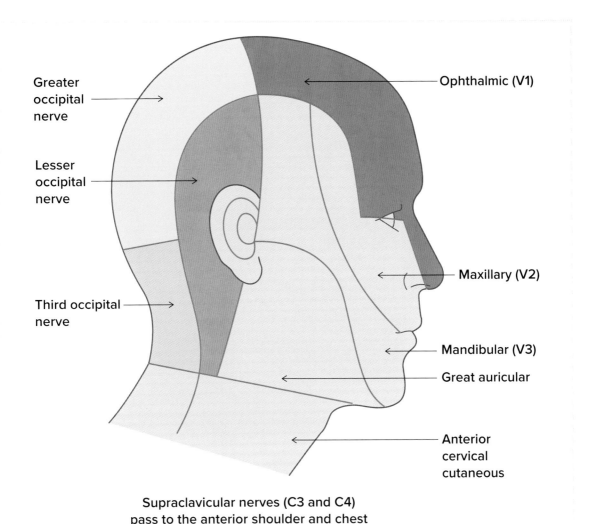

Greater occipital nerve

Lesser occipital nerve

Third occipital nerve

Ophthalmic (V1)

Maxillary (V2)

Mandibular (V3)

Great auricular

Anterior cervical cutaneous

Supraclavicular nerves (C3 and C4)
pass to the anterior shoulder and chest

FIGURE 2.19

High cervical pain referral.

Pain from C1–3 is referred in the distribution of the occipital nerves and the trigeminal nerve to the head and face. Referral of pain to the occipital region follows the distribution of the local cutaneous nerves such as the greater, lesser and third occipital nerves. Pain from occipital neuritis or from injury to the upper cervical joints is referred in the distribution of the occipital nerves.

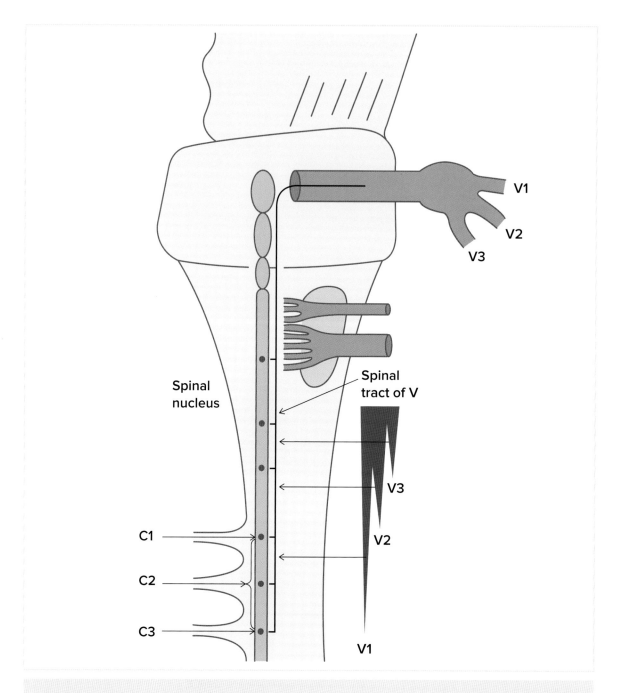

FIGURE 2.20
Pain referral.

Occipitofrontal headaches are common and pain referral to the forehead can be explained by central convergence of the upper three cervical nerves with input from the ophthalmic division of the trigeminal nerve in the spinal tract of V. V1 to V3 lie within the lower brainstem and upper cervical cord. Pain is often referred to the V1 region of the forehead due to the convergence of V1 with C1–3.

CHAPTER 3

ANATOMY OF THE SUBAXIAL SPINE

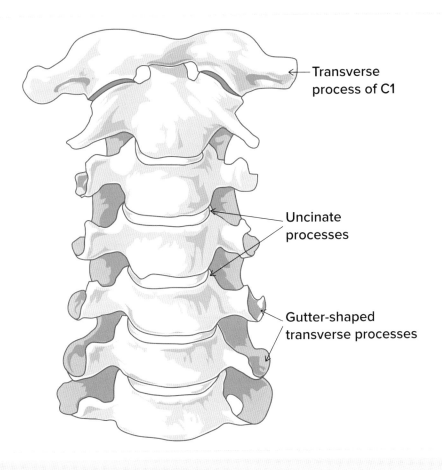

Transverse process of C1

Uncinate processes

Gutter-shaped transverse processes

FIGURE 3.1A

The cervical column viewed from in front.

Viewed from in front the cervical column widens as it descends from C3 to C7. Prominent uncinate processes project upwards at the lateral margins of each vertebral body.

Figure 3.1 continues

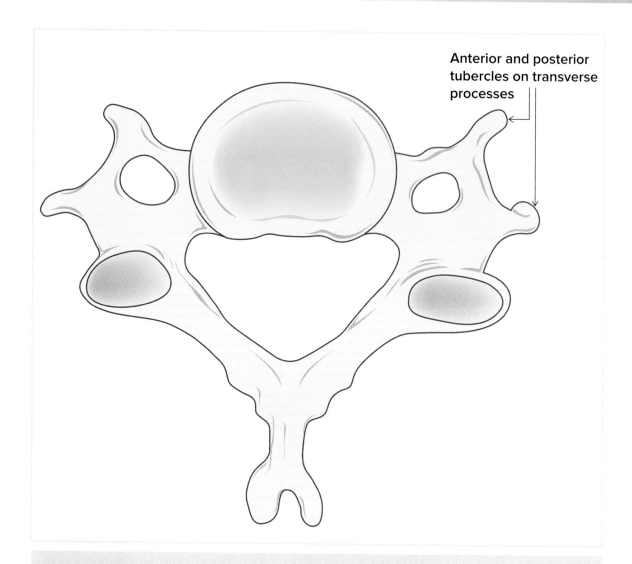

Anterior and posterior
tubercles on transverse
processes

FIGURE 3.1B
Plan view of C3.

The plan view of a 'typical' cervical vertebra, C3, shows its wide triangular spinal canal. The transverse and spinous processes are bifid and the transverse processes are pierced by foramina for the vertebral arteries. The zygapophyseal facets from C2–3 to C4–5 are angled at about 45° to the long axis of the spine.

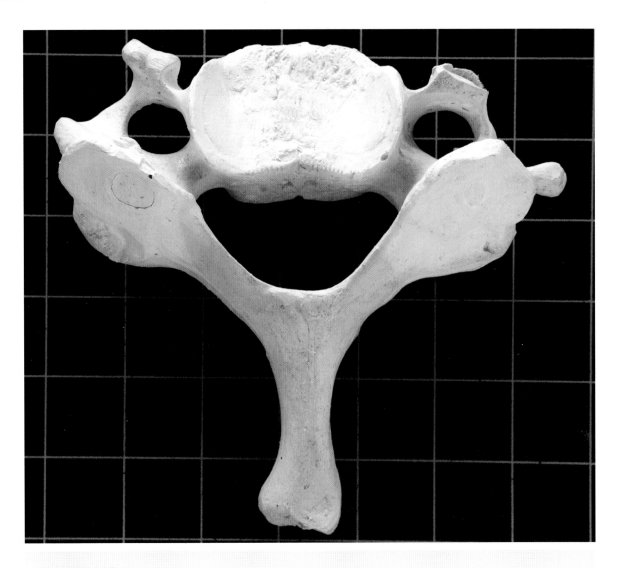

FIGURE 3.1C
Plan view of C6.

The C6 vertebra resembles C3–5 except that it has a longer, easily palpable, non-bifid spinous process and a smaller facet angle (30°). The spinous processes of C7 and T1 are even more prominent and are readily palpable.

The vertebral arteries ascend through all the transverse processes from C6 to C1. The scalenus anterior and scalenus medius arise respectively from the anterior and posterior tubercles on the tips of the transverse processes. The spinal nerves pass out from the spinal canal along gutters in the transverse processes, behind the vertebral arteries, to enter the interscalene plane where they form the brachial plexus. The upper parts of the plexus are palpable in the root of the neck when examining the seated subject from behind and running the fingers around the anterior margin of the scalenus medius.

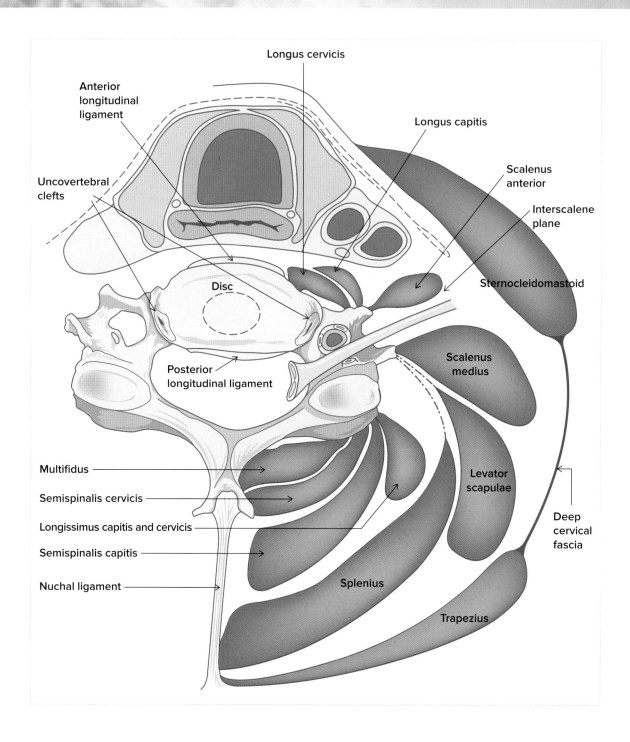

Longus cervicis

Anterior
longitudinal
ligament

Longus capitis

Scalenus
anterior

Interscalene
plane

Uncovertebral
clefts

Disc

Sternocleidomastoid

Posterior
longitudinal ligament

Scalenus
medius

Multifidus

Levator
scapulae

Semispinalis cervicis

Longissimus capitis and cervicis

Deep
cervical
fascia

Semispinalis capitis

Nuchal ligament

Splenius

Trapezius

FIGURE 3.2
A diagram of a transverse section of the neck (at C5–6 level).

Note the close anterior relationship of the cervical spine to the posterior wall of the pharynx and the upper end of the oesophagus. At a higher level than this section, the cervical spine also relates indirectly to the hyoid bone and laryngeal cartilages, parts of which are readily palpable giving successive spinal levels:

- the hyoid cartilage is at the C3 level
- the prominence of the thyroid cartilage is opposite C4–5
- the ring of the cricoid cartilage is at C6 level.

The disc and facet joints are surrounded by muscles: small anterior strap muscles and a large mass of lateral and posterior muscles. Note the marked contrast between the small anterior muscles and the large mass of the posterior muscles.

The nerves that form the brachial plexus pass out of the spinal canal into the interscalene plane. With the subject seated, the upper parts of the brachial plexus can be palpated in this intermuscular plane by sliding the hands round the anterior aspect of the scalenus medius. The discs cannot be readily reached, but the front of the transverse processes can be palpated, close to the discs. In the supine subject, the articular columns of the zygapophyseal joints are readily palpated on each side of the spinous processes.

The loads borne by the cervical spine are much lower than in the lumbar spine, but the cervical spine requires good muscle support from the strong muscles behind and lateral to it. The activity of these muscles imposes loads on the cervical spine. The muscles supporting the upper limb girdle—the trapezius, levator scapulae, rhomboids and sternocleidomastoid—add loading to the neck as they 'suspend' the upper limb from the skull base and the cervical vertebrae. The scalene muscles from the cervical vertebrae to the upper ribs also add loading to the cervical spine when they act as 'guy ropes' to stabilise the spine.

In front on each side of the midline the longus cervicis and longus capitis are closely applied to the anterior vertebral and disc surfaces. Behind the spine, the multifidus and semispinalis cervicis are intimately related to the articular column and individual facet joints as they pass obliquely down from the spinous processes to wrap around the articular columns, one to three segments lower. The semispinalis cervicis and multifidus are covered by the semispinalis capitis, the largest and strongest of the 'vertical' extensors as it ascends to insert behind the foramen magnum. All of these are covered by the oblique fibres of the splenius (the bandage) as it passes up to insert on the superior nuchal line.

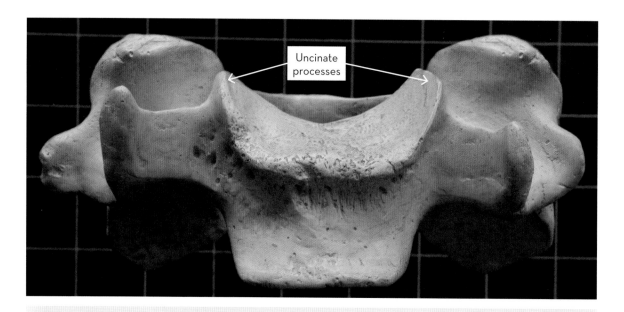

Uncinate
processes

FIGURE 3.3A

The uncinate processes are seen in an anterior view of a cervical vertebra.

The processes project upwards from the lateral margins of the vertebral body, which looks like a chair with side supports.

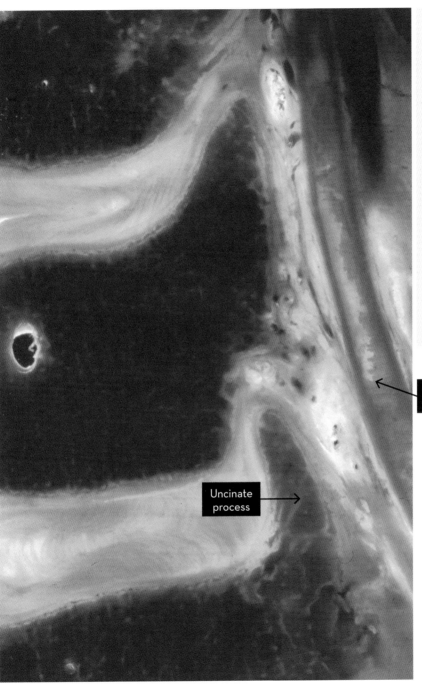

FIGURE 3.3B

A 2.5 mm coronal section of the right half of a young adult spine shows the prominent, sharp nature of these processes.

Lateral to the uncinate processes, the vertebral artery ascends through the transverse foramina of C6 and C5. The tip of each uncus makes a groove for itself in the lower lateral margin of the vertebral body above.

Vertebral artery

Uncinate process

CERVICAL INTERVERTEBRAL DISCS

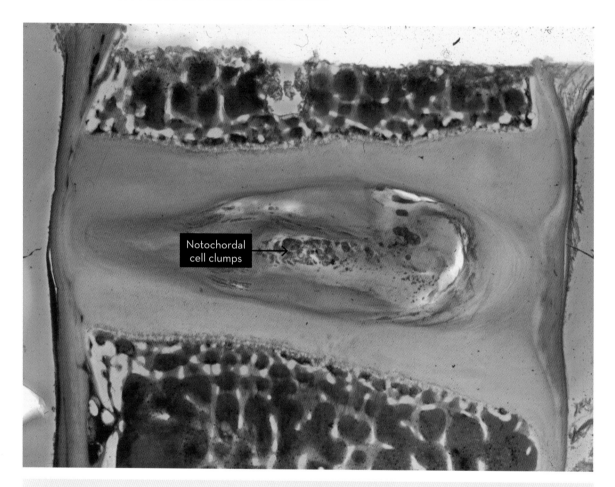

Notochordal cell clumps

FIGURE 3.4A

A normal disc in an infant.

A thin, stained midsagittal section of a low-viscosity nitrocellulose embedded infant cervical disc shows the large nucleus pulposus enclosed by the annulus fibrosus peripherally and by thick cartilage plates above and below. The nucleus still contains notochordal cells, which atrophy during childhood. The inner annulus is fibrocartilaginous and the outer annulus is fibrous. (Anterior is to the right.)

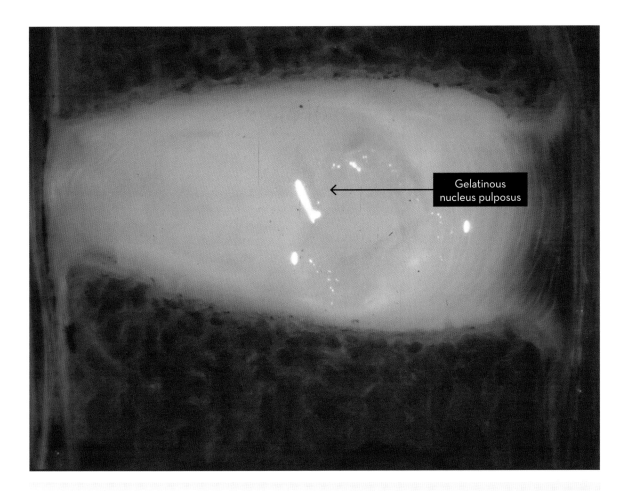

Gelatinous
nucleus pulposus

FIGURE 3.4B
A normal disc in a 19-year-old adult.

A thick, unstained sagittal section of a disc from a 19-year-old who died in a car crash still has a gelatinous nucleus enclosed by an annulus and cartilage plates. The nucleus is swollen with water absorbed from the atmosphere, attracted by the high proteoglycan content of the nucleus. There is blood staining in the anterior annulus.

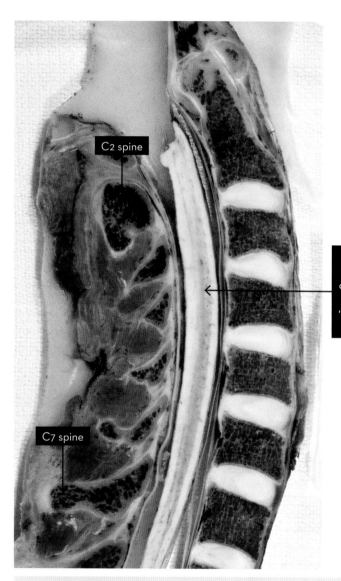

C2 spine

The central 'grey matter' (nerve cells) can be distinguished from the peripheral 'white matter' (nerve fibres or axons).

C7 spine

FIGURE 3.5
A midline section of a normal young cervical spine.

The vertebral bodies are taller posteriorly than anteriorly, conforming to the normal lordotic posture of the cervical spine. The normal dura and spinal cord are in situ. Disc thickness contributes a higher proportion of the column length than in other regions, reflecting greater cervical mobility. The C2, C7 and T1 spines are the most prominent and easily palpable; the bifid short spines of C3 to C5 are also palpable.

In two separate studies we measured mid-disc thickness midway between the anterior and posterior margins of each disc in two different groups of cervical spines, in discs where there was no evidence of trauma (Head, 1995; Taylor, 1996). The distance from the vertebral endplate above to the endplate below in young adults was about 7 mm on average, with a standard deviation of 1 mm. Average disc thickness decreased significantly with ageing into the 70s (see Chapter 4).

Figure 3.6 illustrates a lower lumbar disc. Cervical discs in adolescents and young adults resemble lumbar discs in their structure. But in early adult life, cervical discs begin to change and they become quite different from lumbar discs.

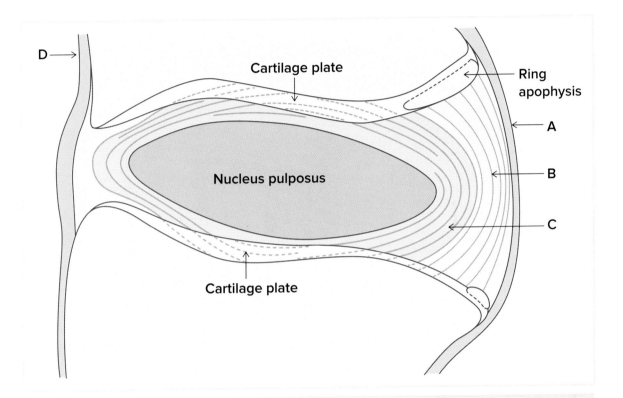

FIGURE 3.6
Diagram of a midline sagittal section of a young adult intervertebral disc.

The anterior longitudinal ligament **(A)** covers the anterior annulus fibrosus, which has two parts: the outer collagenous annulus **(B)**, which passes from the vertebral rim above to the vertebral rim below; and the inner fibrocartilaginous annulus **(C)**, which is continuous above and below with the cartilage plates and forms an envelope that contains the gelatinous nucleus pulposus of the young person. The posterior longitudinal ligament **(D)** covers the surface of the posterior annulus. The vertebral rim is formed by the fusion of the ring apophysis with the vertebral body in adolescence. The outer collagenous annulus is the most vulnerable to injury on extension: it usually tears at its junction with the vertebral rim. The longer fibres of the two longitudinal ligaments are resilient and can stretch without tearing.

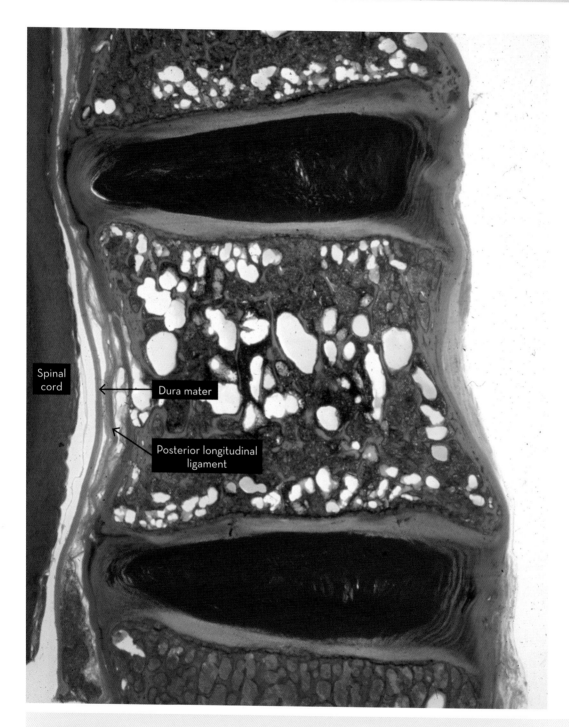

FIGURE 3.7A

A 100-micron stained sagittal section of cervical discs from a 17-year-old youth.

The midsagittal section shows normal C5–6 and C6–7 discs. The nucleus pulposus stains red. The cartilage plates above and below it stain light green.

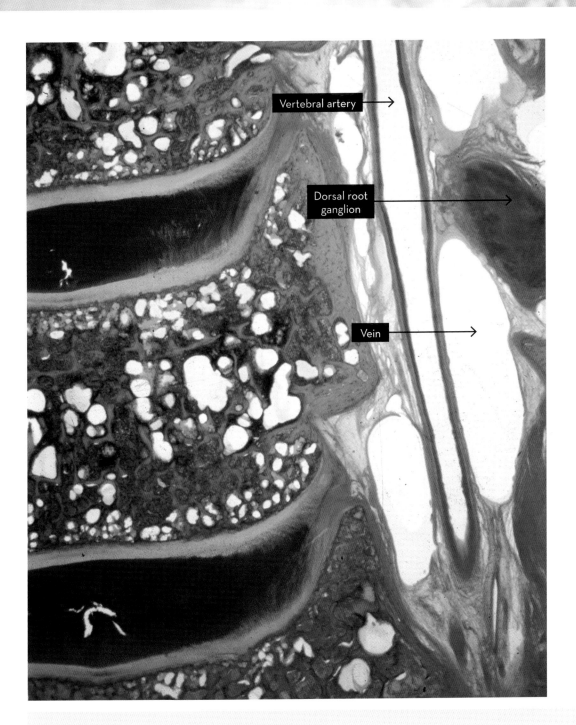

FIGURE 3.7B
A coronal section from the same individual as in Figure 3.7A.

This coronal section shows the left half of the C4–5 and 5–6 discs with the vertebral vessels alongside. The vertebral artery lies between two empty vertebral veins with a large oval dorsal root ganglion lateral to the blood vessels.

Figure 3.7 continues

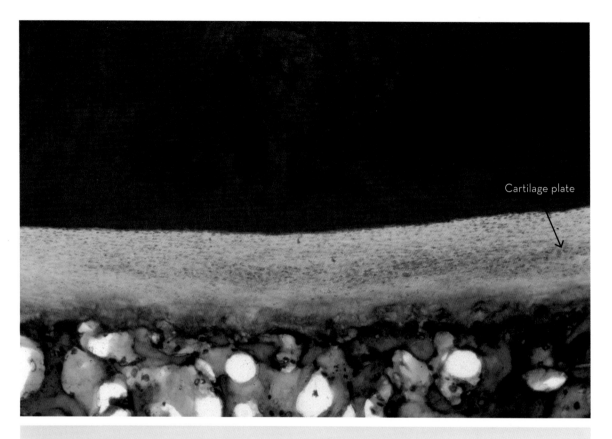

Cartilage plate

FIGURE 3.7C

Detail of the normal cartilage plate (C6–7) that separates the vascular vertebral spongiosa (green) from the avascular nucleus pulposus (red).

Haematoxylin deeply stains the proteoglycan-rich nucleus pulposus. The annulus and the bone stain with the acidic 'light green'.

ZYGAPOPHYSEAL FACET JOINTS

Facet orientation in the sagittal plane. The zygapophyseal facet joints of the young adult are oriented at an average of 45° to the long axis of the spine except at the lower two levels where they are closer to 30° to the long axis of the spine. In children they are oriented closer to the horizontal plane than the adult facets; this gives children a greater range of mobility as the rotational movements are accompanied by increased translation, which involves shearing forces in the young discs. The approximate 45° facet orientation means that axial rotation and side bending are coupled in the subaxial cervical spine but central nervous control adjusts for this so that looking to the side is not normally accompanied by looking downwards.

Facet orientation in the axial plane. Viewed from above (see Figure 3.1B and C) the zygapophyseal facet joint planes are very close to the coronal plane, but at C3 the posterior-facing facets are angled slightly inwards and backwards, while at C6 they are angled slightly outwards and backwards as in the thoracic spine. Milne (1993) measured these angles in a large osteological series and related the inward slant at C2–3 to the reduced range of axial rotation at that level compared to levels above and below. C2–3 is relatively stiff compared to the wide range of movement in the two segments above and the three segments below. This may increase the loading of its joints in forced rotation or injury.

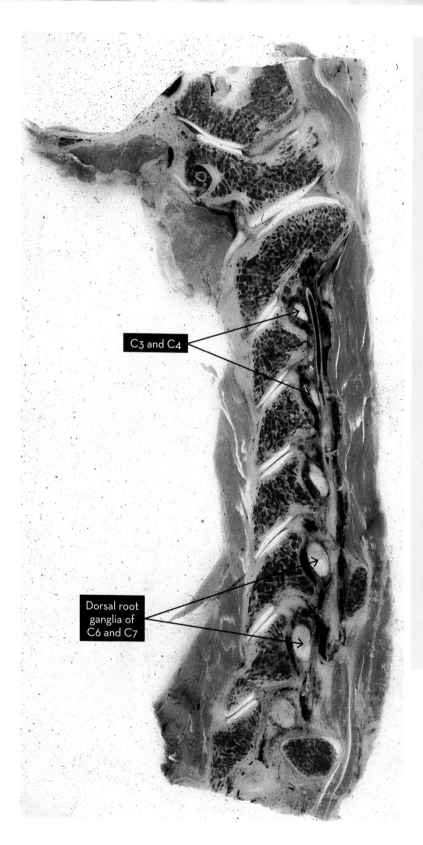

C3 and C4

Dorsal root
ganglia of
C6 and C7

FIGURE 3.8A
A sagittal section through the facet joints and articular column in a 20-year-old man.

The section shows a regular articular column with normal facet orientation. In front of the articular column the vertebral artery passes vertically upwards and the spinal nerves exit from the intervertebral foramina, passing out between the articular column and the vertebral artery in hollows on the front of the articular column. The C5 to C8 nerves that form the brachial plexus are much larger than the nerves of C3 to C4. The C0–1 and C1–2 lateral joints are on a more anterior plane than the zygapophyseal facets. The head of the first rib is sectioned at the lower end of the section.

The facet joints show the typical adult orientation at about 45° to the long axis of the spine. The vertebral artery is very small on this side (vertebral arteries are often asymmetrical). Most of the posterior muscles have been removed.

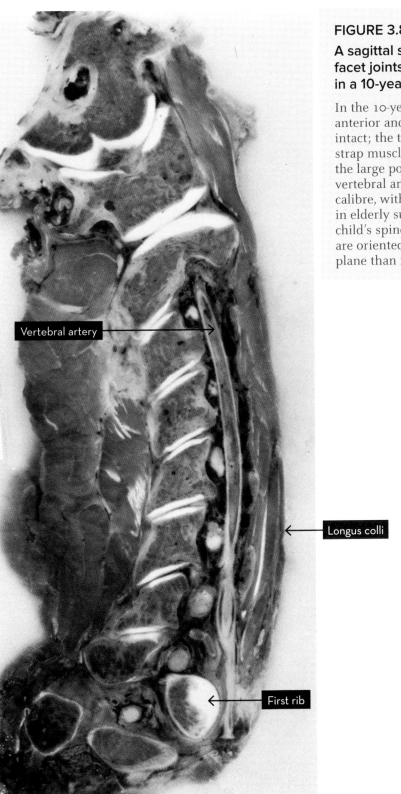

Vertebral artery

Longus colli

First rib

FIGURE 3.8B

A sagittal section through the facet joints and articular column in a 10-year-old child.

In the 10-year-old most of the anterior and posterior muscles are intact; the thin anterior longus colli strap muscles in front contrast with the large posterior muscles. The vertebral artery has a normal regular calibre, without the tortuosity seen in elderly subjects. The facets in this child's spine, as in most children, are oriented closer to the horizontal plane than in the adult spine.

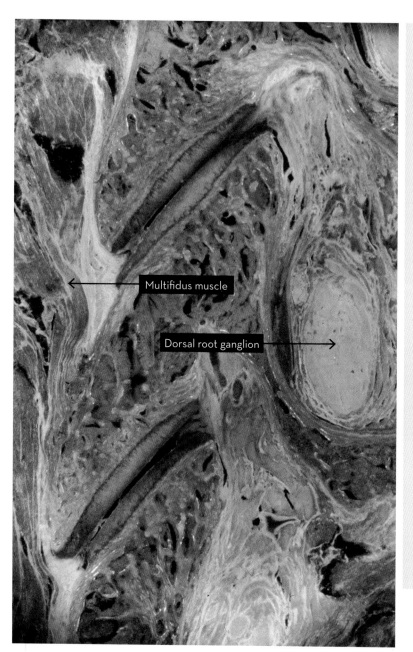

Multifidus muscle

Dorsal root ganglion

FIGURE 3.9A

A sagittal section of normal synovial facet joints from a 35-year-old man (dark ground illumination).

A sagittal section of C5–6 and C6–7. Anterior to the joints a large dorsal root ganglion lies in a hollow in the front of the articular column. Behind the joints, the multifidus muscle descends obliquely from the spinous processes above to insert into the articular column. Its deep fibres, reinforced by the semispinalis cervicis, enclose and are intimately related to the posterior surface of the joint as they cover the inferior joint recess to insert into the articular column below the joint margin. The deepest fibres of the multifidus muscle are lined by the joint synovial membrane. Vascular synovial folds move freely in and out of the joint during normal movement. No separate fibrous capsule is visible.

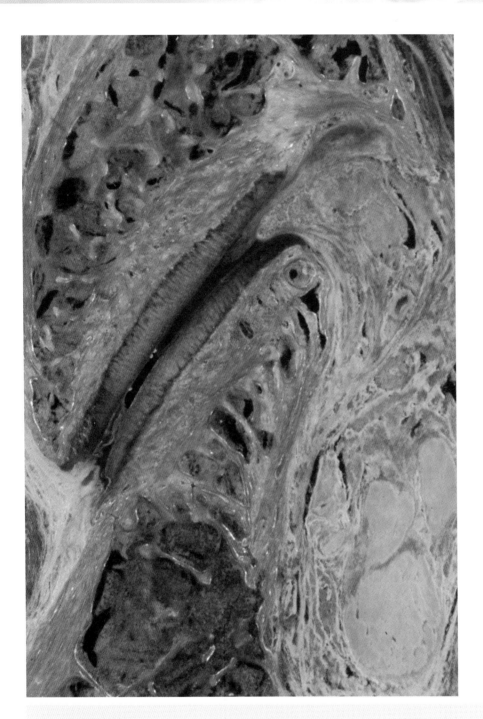

FIGURE 3.9B
A sagittal section of the C6–7 facet joint in closer view.

The smooth articular cartilages (dark blue) are supported by compact subchondral bone plates. The cancellous bone network of the articular column has bone marrow in its interstices. The section shows the upper synovial fold projecting into the joint between the articular margins.

MOVEMENT

The Dutch radiologist Penning performed classical studies of the cervical spine including radiographic measurement of segmental range of movement (ROM) (Penning, 1978). The lower ROM at C2–3 probably relates to its lower interfacet angle as described above (page 53 and Figure 3.1B on page 40). Milne (1993) reviewed 17 published studies of sagittal ROM and published the mean values for these studies, as shown in Table 3.1.

TABLE 3.1 Values for sagittal and axial ROM			
	Sagittal range (Penning)	Rotation right + left (Penning)	Sagittal range (Milne)
C0–1	30°	70°	
C1–2	30°		
C2–3	12°		11.1
C3–4	18°		14.8
C4–5	20°	70°	17.4
C5–6	20°		19.8
C6–7	18°		16.4

The nature of segmental movement depends on facet orientation. The centre of motion reflects the influence of the facet angles on movement. At C2–3, C3–4 and C4–5, with facet angles of about 45°, the centre of motion is well below the discs; at C5–6 and C6–7 with facet angles of about 30°, the centre of motion is close below the discs. Therefore, the upper discs are subjected to greater shearing forces in all types of rotation; there is less shear but greater ROM in the C5–6 disc.

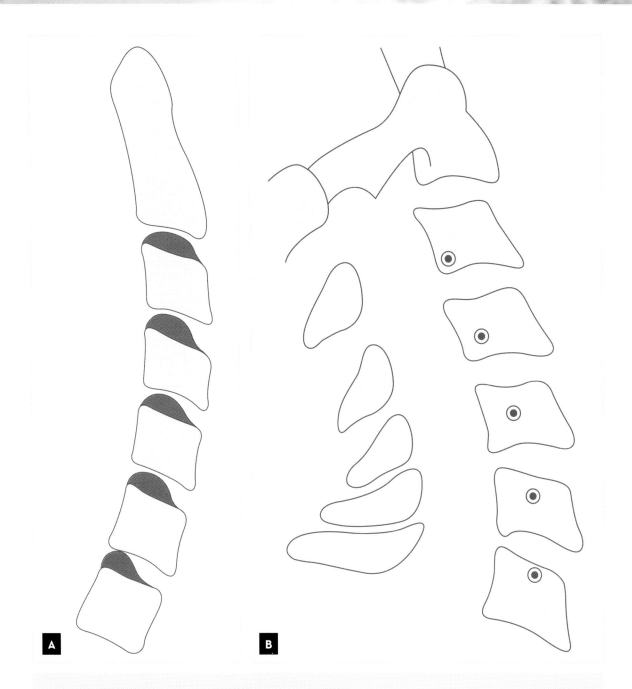

FIGURE 3.10A and B

Penning calculated the centre of motion at each subaxial level and described segmental variation in the position of the uncus.

These images show the position of the uncus at different levels (red) **(A)** and the position of the centres of motion **(B)**. The uncus is lateral at upper levels and posterolateral at lower levels. The uncus forms the anteromedial boundary of the intervertebral foramen and its posterolateral position at lower cervical levels is very close to the emerging spinal nerves.

SPINAL NERVES AND THE BRACHIAL PLEXUS

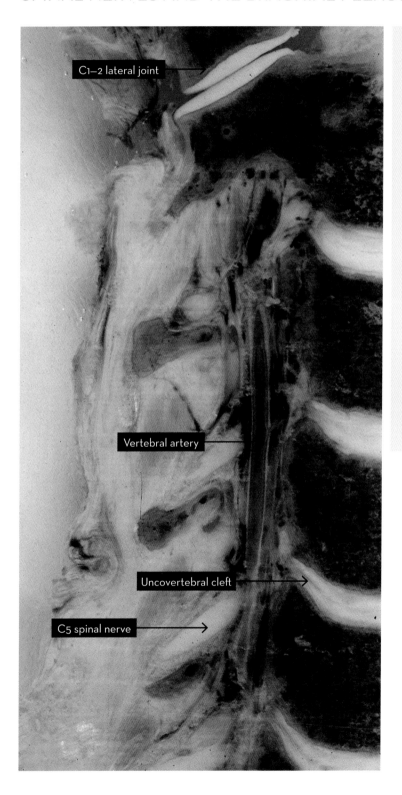

C1–2 lateral joint

Vertebral artery

Uncovertebral cleft

C5 spinal nerve

FIGURE 3.11A

A coronal section of the right half of the cervical spine from C1 to C5.

The vertebral artery ascends from C6 and parts of the lower spinal nerves emerge from behind it as they descend laterally towards the brachial plexus. This coronal section of a 29-year-old man shows the straight course of the vertebral artery and parts of the C4, C5 and C6 spinal nerves. Lateral fissures can be seen in the discs in the uncovertebral regions of the lower discs. At their origins, the cervical nerves lie above their respective vertebrae but the thoracic nerves exit below their respective vertebrae, so the 'extra' cervical nerve between C7 and T1 is named C8.

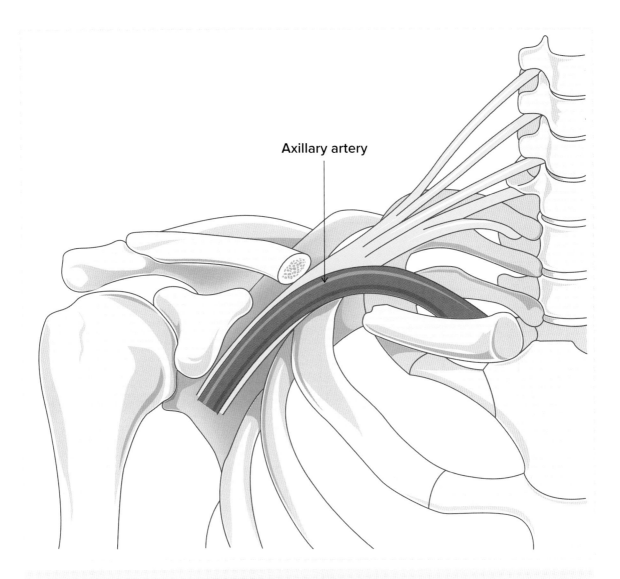

Axillary artery

FIGURE 3.11B
The formation of the brachial plexus.

The middle portion of the clavicle is removed to show the plexus descending with the axillary artery into the axilla. C5 and C6 join to form the upper trunk, C7 forms the middle trunk and C8 and T1 form the lower trunk. The upper parts of the plexus are palpable in the interscalene plane (see Figure 3.2).

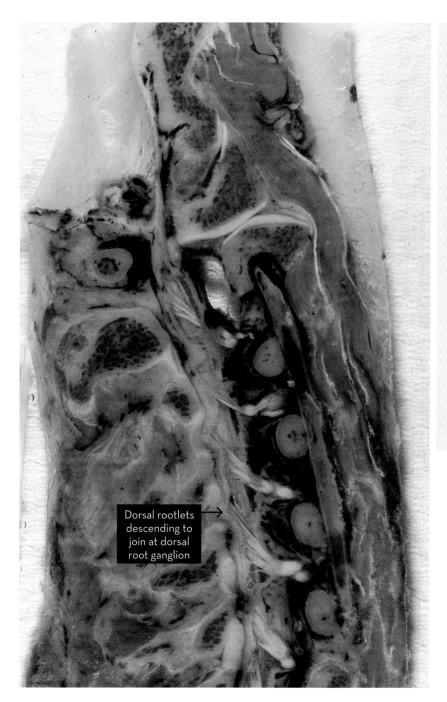

Dorsal rootlets
descending to
join at dorsal
root ganglion

FIGURE 3.12
The early course of the sensory roots of cervical spinal nerves in a thick sagittal section.

Dorsal rootlets arise in neat linear series from the back of the spinal cord; they descend laterally and forwards, multiple rootlets joining to form single dorsal roots at the dorsal root ganglia. The dorsal root ganglia lie above and behind the smaller motor roots, both surrounded by small veins in the lateral recess of the spinal canal and the intervertebral foramina.

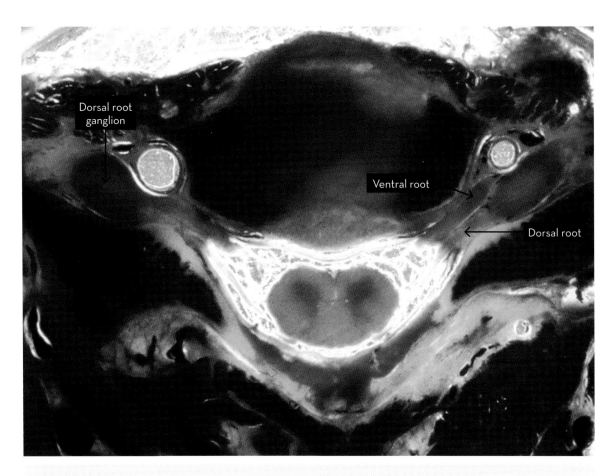

FIGURE 3.13
Origins of spinal nerves in a transverse section from a 72-year-old woman.

This dissecting room specimen shows the dorsal and ventral roots passing obliquely forwards and laterally. The dorsal roots pass more obliquely forwards than the ventral roots and are therefore subject to stretch in extension as well as in side bending. The large dorsal root ganglia are in direct contact with the vertebral arteries as they pass out between the uncus and the articular column.

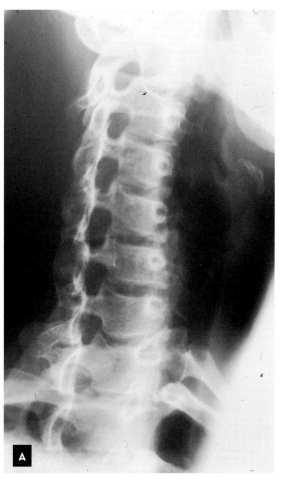

A

FIGURE 3.14A and B
Oblique views show the intervertebral foramina and their boundaries.

The size of the dorsal nerve root in the diagram **(B)** is smaller than actual size; the lower cervical dorsal root ganglia normally almost fill the foramina. The proximity of the uncus to the nerve roots is of primary importance in relation to age changes, when growth of uncovertebral osteophytes into the foramen may impinge on the nerves, mainly on the larger dorsal root or its ganglion, so that symptoms are predominantly sensory.

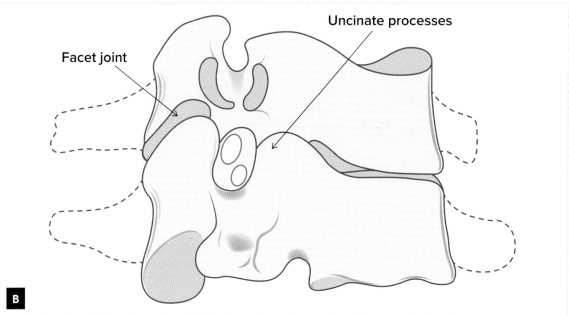

B

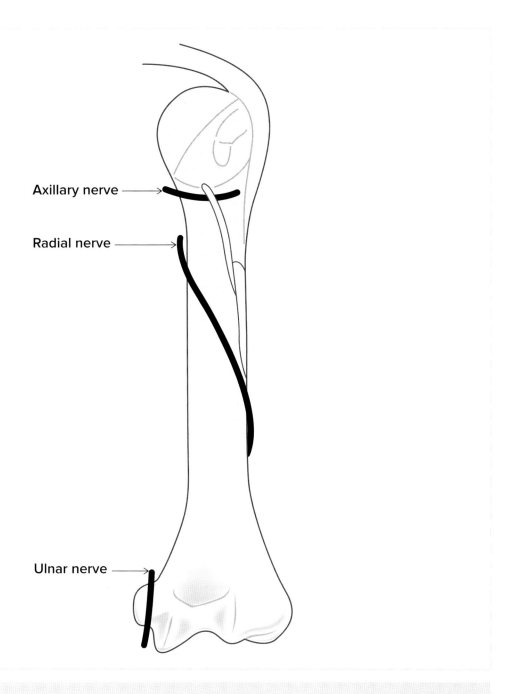

FIGURE 3.15

Palpable terminal branches of the brachial plexus.

Three major nerves have a close relationship with the posterior aspect of the humerus: the axillary nerve (C5, 6), the radial nerve (C5–T1) and the ulnar nerve (C8, T1). The median nerve is palpable in the cubital fossa medial to the brachial artery. These nerves can be tested by stretching them (Elvey, 1986).

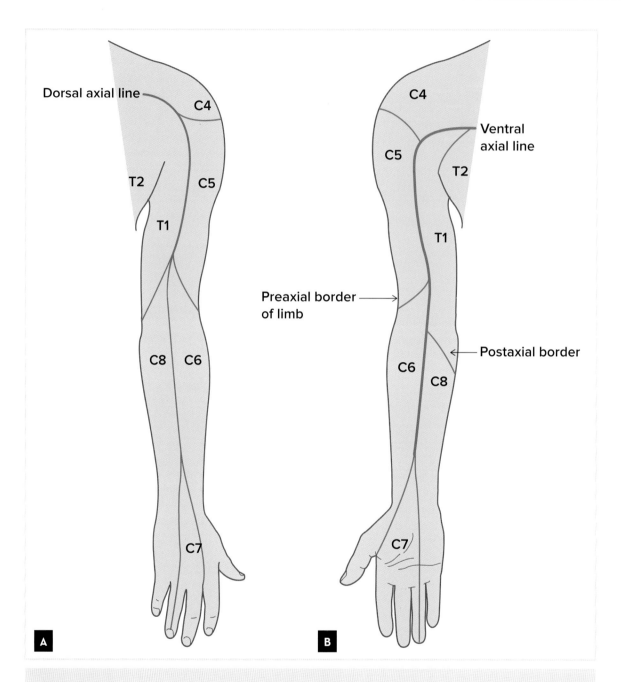

FIGURE 3.16

Upper limb dermatomes: segmental innervation to the skin.

Anterior **(A)** and posterior **(B)** views of typical dermatomal patterns of skin innervation. These patterns are useful when judging pain referral from the neck. They are reasonably consistent between individuals but with minor variations. The pattern is determined by growth of the fetal limb bud, with innervation being 'drawn out' as the limb bud grows. C4 supplies the top of the shoulder; C5 to T1 are derived from the brachial plexus.

SEGMENTAL INNERVATION AND PATTERNS OF PAIN REFERRAL

Spinal nerves innervate skin dermatomes and muscle myotomes. When a structure (e.g. a joint) is injured, pain is referred to the corresponding dermatome or, less often, there is loss of power in its myotome; for example, if the C5–6 facet joint or disc is injured, the patient will usually fill in an area corresponding to the C6 dermatome on a pain diagram (Figure 3.17). Thus a knowledge of upper limb dermatomes and myotomes is essential for a logical and accurate diagnostic assessment of a patient's pain.

Pain may also be referred in the distribution of cutaneous or sensory muscle innervation; for example, to the anterior chest from C3–4 disc to the area supplied by the supraclavicular nerves. Pain has been shown to be referred from the anterior surface of cervical discs to the interscapular area (Cloward, 1959).

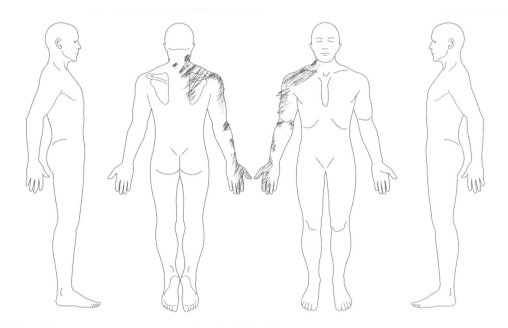

FIGURE 3.17
A patient's pain diagram showing C6 radiculopathy.

A knowledge of normal segmental innervation is useful in finding the source of a patient's pain. Aprill and Bogduk (1990) found a close relationship between a patient's pain diagram and the eventual diagnosis of the site of injury.

Sensation   Motor

C5

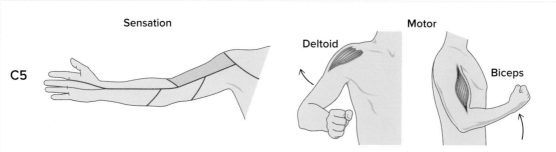

C5 innervates the deltoid and biceps and gives sensation to the dermatome over the deltoid.

C6

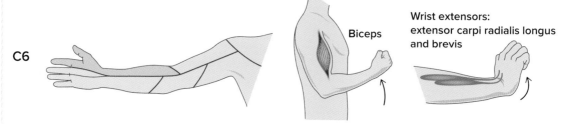

C6 innervates the dermatome over the lateral forearm and hand and innervates the wrist extensors.

C7

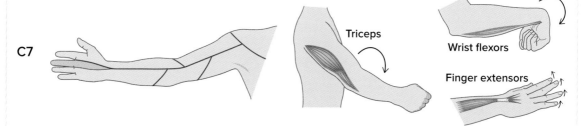

C7 innervates the small dermatome over the middle finger plus the triceps, wrist flexors and finger extensors.

C8

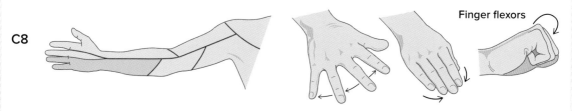

C8 supplies the dermatome of the medial hand and forearm plus the finger flexors.

T1

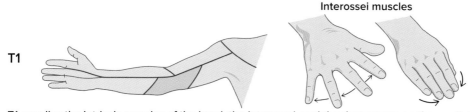

T1 supplies the intrinsic muscles of the hand, the interossei, and the dermatome on the medial upper arm.

FIGURE 3.18
Segmental innervation.

This shows the dermatomal and myotomal innervation through the brachial plexus. These are used to test for any deficits from injury or other pathology. The biceps reflex (C5), the brachioradialis reflex (C6) and the triceps reflex (C7) are also used to test the integrity of the C5, C6 and C7 sensory and motor connections through the spinal cord.

The cutaneous innervation of the head and shoulders and its relationship to pain referral from higher spinal segments is shown in Figure 2.19 on page 37.

Dwyer and colleagues (1990) tested the pain referral pattern from facet joints by injecting each other and produced a chart showing the wide overlap between pain from adjacent facets (Figure 3.19). A Japanese study of 61 patients by Fukui and colleagues (1996) charted a similar but more complex map of the sites of pain referral from the facets.

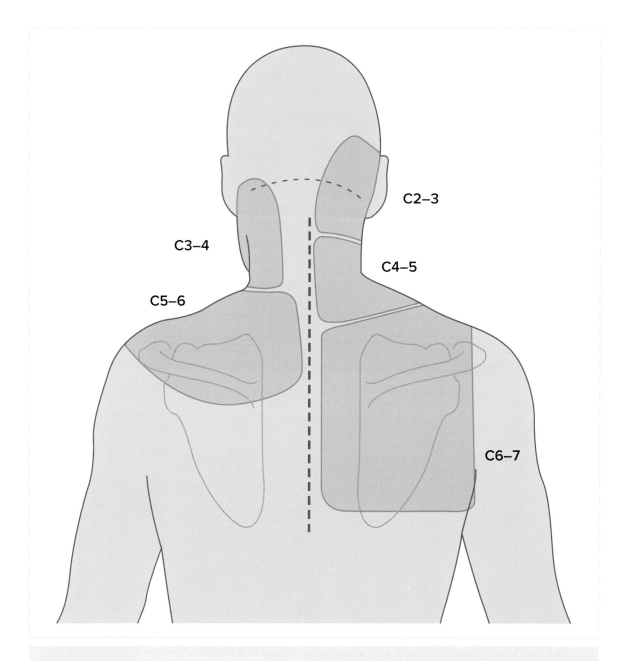

FIGURE 3.19
Pain referral patterns from facet joints.

THE COURSE OF THE VERTEBRAL ARTERY IN THE NECK

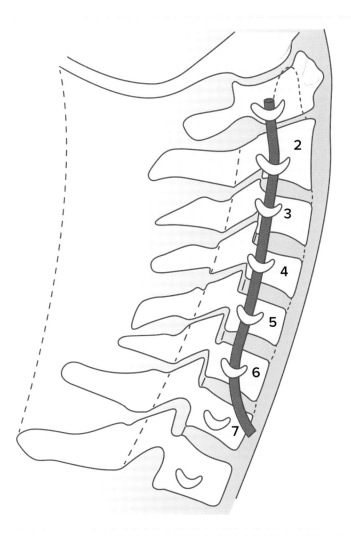

FIGURE 3.20

The course of the vertebral artery from C6 to C1.

This branch of the subclavian artery arises in the root of the neck and passes up through the transverse processes from C6 to C1 to pierce the dura at the foramen magnum and join the circle of Willis to supply the hindbrain. Vertebral veins occupy the C7 transverse foramen.

It also supplies the cervical spine and the cervical spinal cord. An anterior spinal artery supplies the cord's central grey matter and two smaller posterior spinal arteries supply the outer layers of the cord (white matter). These spinal arteries are reinforced segmentally by small radicular branches. Sympathetic grey rami communicantes from the cervicothoracic (stellate) ganglion form a plexus around the vertebral artery and follow it to join roots of the brachial plexus (C7 to T1). Other sympathetic nerves for the brachial plexus arise from the middle cervical ganglion to join C5 and C6.

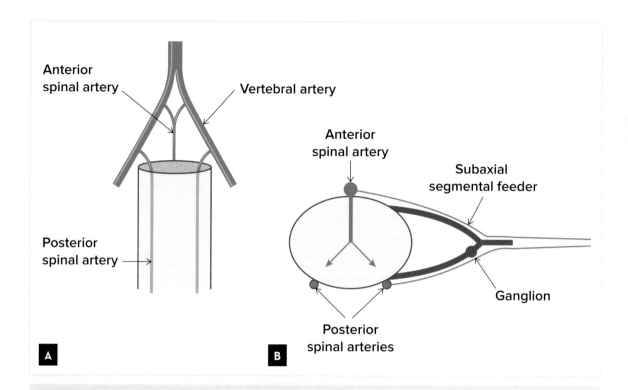

FIGURE 3.21A and B

Blood supply of the cervical spinal cord.

(A) Three spinal arteries are derived from the vertebral arteries, one anterior and two posterior. The larger anterior spinal artery supplies the central grey matter; the smaller posterior spinal arteries supply the outer white matter. **(B)** At a number of subaxial cervical levels, 'feeders' from the vertebral arteries pass as radicular branches along the nerve roots to reinforce the spinal arteries.

CHAPTER 4

AGE CHANGES IN THE CERVICAL SPINE: THE CERVICAL DISCS

Age changes in the cervical spine predominantly affect the intervertebral discs. Disc changes occur at a much earlier age in the subaxial cervical spine than in other regions (Taylor, Twomey & Levander, 2000). Fortunately, the synovial joints of the upper two cervical segments are generally well preserved in older people. Changes in the zygapophyseal facet joints appear to occur later than the disc changes, perhaps in response to the altered biomechanics from disc degeneration and loss of disc thickness.

The continuum of age changes begins when the uncinate processes grow upwards from the lateral margins of the vertebral bodies in late childhood. The growth of the uncus significantly narrows the lateral intervertebral gap by puberty, then the shearing forces accompanying movements cause uncovertebral clefts to appear in the narrowed, lateral margins of the discs. Shearing forces in the discs of the highly mobile cervical segments are facilitated by the 45° facet orientation. The shearing forces accompany rotations in the sagittal, coronal and axial planes. The discs of young adults begin to show disc fissuring, spreading from the uncovertebral clefts into the centres of the discs, so that by the mid-30s the nucleus is often fissured and is no longer enclosed by a complete annulus and cartilage plate envelope. The typical young adult arrangement in other spinal regions is of a nucleus enclosed by an intact envelope of annulus and cartilage plates. This no longer applies in cervical discs and the nucleus itself becomes degraded and is no longer recognisable as the fluid gelatinous nucleus pulposus of the 19-year-old disc.

Potentially damaging degenerative changes usually do not begin until late middle life. First, the central discs become 'scarred' by progressive increases in collagen content. Then, as the discs lose height, the uncinate processes begin to be deflected outwards as uncovertebral osteophytes. These morbid anatomical changes in the discs principally affect C4–5, C5–6 and C6–7. These are normally the most mobile segments of the subaxial spine, so their degenerative changes are accompanied by increasing neck stiffness in late middle age and old age. Concurrent osteoporotic changes in the thoracic spine of old age lead to increased thoracic kyphosis, requiring the cervical spine to adopt an increasingly lordotic posture. This severely limits the available range of remaining extension from the new lordotic posture. Normal movements such as looking up become increasingly difficult in elderly people, who may complain of dizziness in attempted full neck extension (Yukuwa et al., 2012).

By the age of 80, it is common to see spontaneous interbody fusions across the lower cervical resorbed discs. The resultant lower cervical stiffness makes the affected people vulnerable to life threatening trauma to upper cervical levels from simple falls forward with anterior head impact and forced extension.

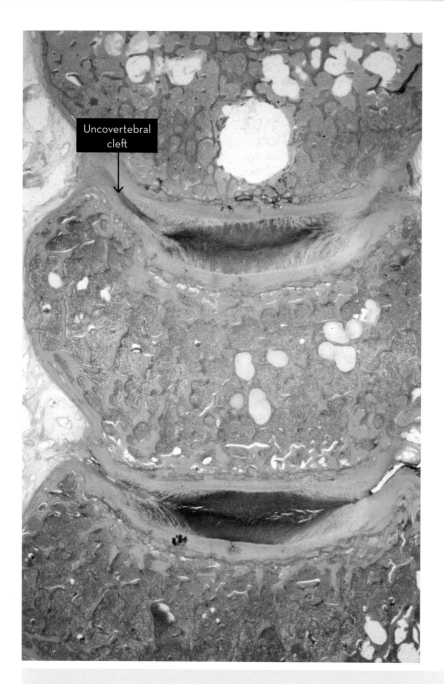

Uncovertebral cleft

FIGURE 4.1A

A coronal section of cervical discs from a 14-year-old girl shows the newly developed uncovertebral clefts.

The uncovertebral clefts are bounded above and below by cartilage plates. These clefts are not true joints, although they resemble joints in some respects; all true joints develop prenatally. The uncovertebral clefts develop at puberty in the narrowed outer part of the disc, between the upwardly growing uncus and the vertebra above.

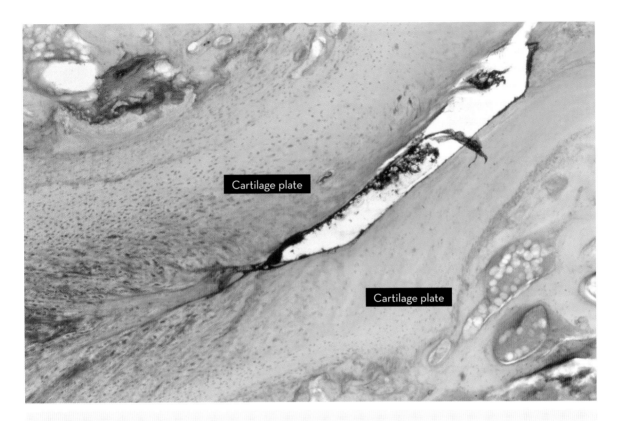

FIGURE 4.1B
A close view of an uncovertebral cleft in a 14-year-old female.

The cleft is bounded by cartilage above and below. The dehydration process in preparation has widened the gap.

FISSURING OF CERVICAL DISCS

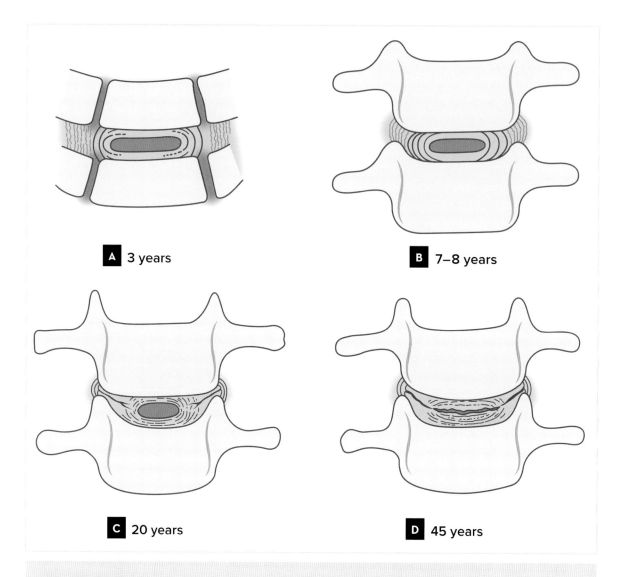

A | 3 years

B | 7–8 years

C | 20 years

D | 45 years

FIGURE 4.2A–D

Stages of disc fissuring.

(A) At 3 years of age the vertebral arches are still separated from the central vertebral bodies by cartilage growth plates. **(B)** At 7–8 years the uncus is actively growing to narrow the lateral intervertebral space. **(C)** By 20 years the uncovertebral clefts are beginning to spread medially as fissures into the annulus. **(D)** By 45 years most people show complete fissuring across the posterior half of the disc and there is no longer a central enclosed nucleus pulposus. Only the two longitudinal ligaments and the anterior annulus are intact.

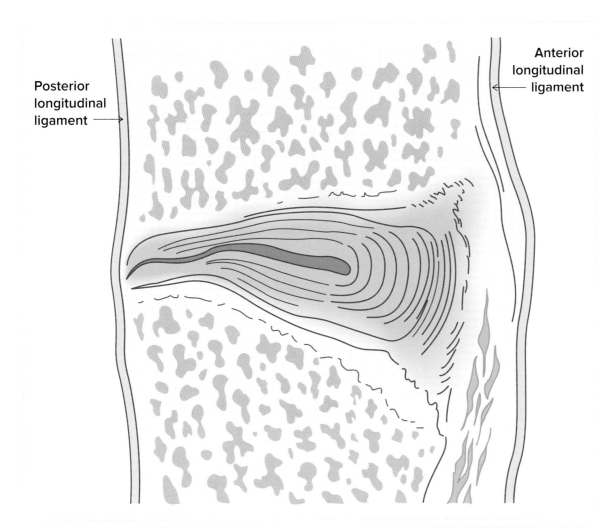

Posterior longitudinal ligament

Anterior longitudinal ligament

FIGURE 4.3
A diagram based on sagittal sections of cadaver discs from elderly subjects.

There is no intact envelope enclosing a nucleus pulposus; there is therefore no nucleus and only the anterior annulus and the two longitudinal ligaments are intact.

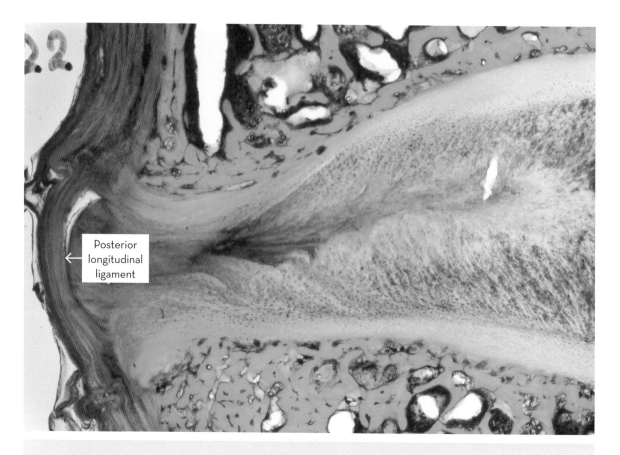

Posterior longitudinal ligament

FIGURE 4.4A

A 100-micron stained section shows the effects of shearing with scarring.

A midsagittal section of C4–5 in a 22-year-old man: green staining demonstrates collagen formation, representing the pre-fissuring stage of scarring due to shearing forces. The intact posterior longitudinal ligament covers the posterior annulus fibrosus.

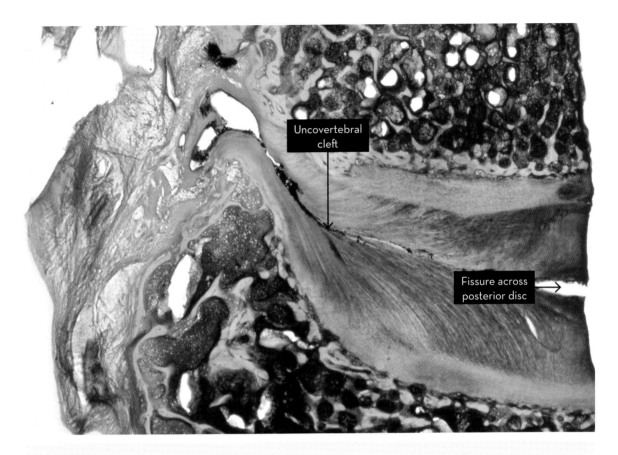

Uncovertebral cleft

Fissure across posterior disc

FIGURE 4.4B

A 100-micron stained coronal section shows the effects of shearing with the development of fissures.

A coronal section of the right half of the C3–4 disc from the same 22-year-old man as in Figure 4.4A shows a complete transverse fissure from the uncovertebral cleft through the centre of the disc. Indian ink, injected into the centre of the disc before fixation and processing, has tracked to the uncovertebral cleft, which is an atypical adventitious joint. The fissures are more clearly visible in low-viscosity nitrocellulose 100-micron sections than in thick 2.5 mm sections. The slight contraction artefact during the dehydration stage of low-viscosity nitrocellulose processing makes the fissuring more obvious, but the spread of Indian ink before processing confirms the real presence of the fissure.

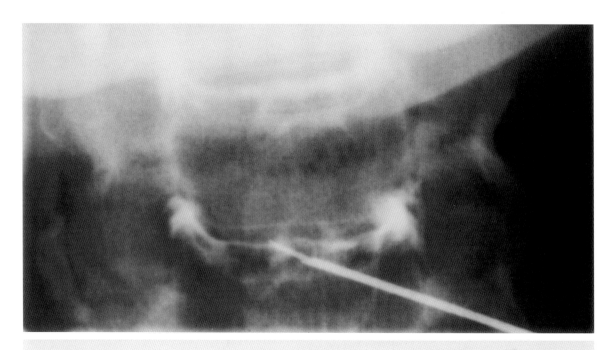

FIGURE 4.5A

Discography demonstrates the extent of fissuring in a young adult patient.

Centrally injected contrast has spread transversely to accumulate in both uncovertebral clefts.

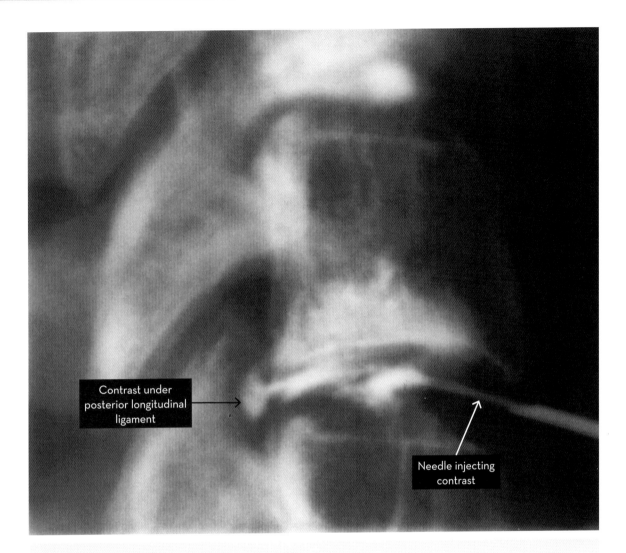

Figure 4.5B

Discography demonstrates the extent of fissuring in the same patient as in Figure 4.5A.

Posteriorly, contrast has spread through the fissure in the posterior annulus to balloon out the intact posterior longitudinal ligament. The fissure is about midway between the two vertebral endplates.

Discograms performed in our autopsy spines demonstrated a difference between the 20-year-old age group and individuals in their 30s. In 61% of discs (11 of 18 discs) of individuals aged 19–21 years, contrast was contained within an enclosed nucleus by an intact annulus, whereas in 76% of discs (31 of 41 discs) in subjects aged 22 to 42 years (average age 32 years) discograms showed leakage through posterolateral annular fissures to the uncovertebral clefts (Milne, 1993). Tondury (1959), in a classical study of 150 cadaver cervical spines ranging from 20 to 90 years of age, described the spread of fissures through the centres of discs in early middle age. In addition, the eminent spinal surgeon Carl Hirsch showed that fissuring was common in young adult discograms (Hirsch, Schazowitz & Galante, 1967).

DISC CHANGES IN SUBJECTS FROM 30 TO 80 YEARS OF AGE

Loss of disc height

In our study we performed two measurement studies of disc height (MDH) in midline sections in two different series of our sections from different groups of uninjured individuals. Both studies found statistically significant losses in MDH, measured from vertebral endplate to vertebral endplate, midway between the anterior and posterior disc margins. At C4–5, C5–6 and C6–7, there was a 20% loss of MDH comparing adults over 60 years of age with adults in their 20s; C2–3 and C7–T1 discs showed no significant age change (Head, 1995; Taylor, 1996). However, the age-related reductions in mean values of MDH do not tell the whole story. The much greater standard deviations in the older age groups reflect a wide range of variation in elderly discs. Values in young adults were all within a narrow band, but the MDH in elderly subjects varied from 0 to 'normal'.

A descriptive study of disc degeneration in 100 uninjured autopsy spines (Taylor, 1996) compared changes observed in subjects aged 60 to 86 years of age with discs in young adults. Most changes were in C4–5, C5–6 and C6–7 discs: 12% of C4–5, 31% of C5–6 and 31% of C6–7 showed either 50% loss of disc height or, less often, complete disc resorption with interbody fusion. We cannot claim that the subjects were entirely 'unselected': we may have seen a higher proportion of degenerate spines than in the general population. But there is ample evidence of both structural loss of disc height and marked reduction in range of motion with ageing.

Our findings of MDH loss are supported by more recent studies which found significant reductions in disc height in C5–6 and C6–7 when comparing 60–70-year-old subjects to 20-year-old subjects; functional studies have also found an average loss of 35% of sagittal range of motion from young adult life to old age (Yukuwa et al., 2012; Zejda & Bartolomiej, 2003; Okada, Masumoto, Fujiwara & Toyama, 2011).

Loss of disc height is associated with the formation of uncovertebral osteophytes, which may impinge upon the spinal nerves, the vertebral arteries and/or the spinal cord.

Uncovertebral osteophytes and their effects

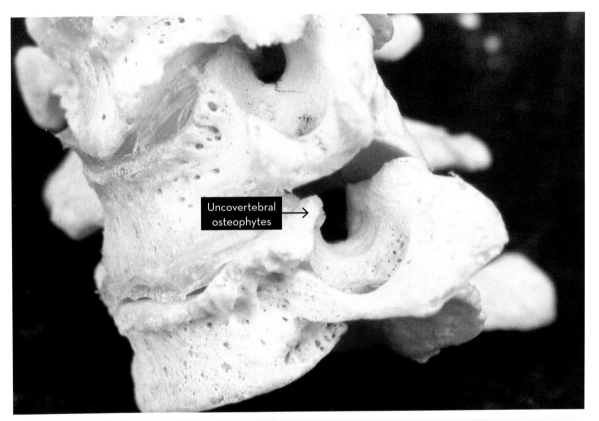

FIGURE 4.6

Disc degeneration.

An oblique view of lower cervical vertebrae from an elderly subject (from the dissecting room) shows a lower intervertebral foramen constricted by uncovertebral osteophytes due to disc degeneration.

Effects on nerves

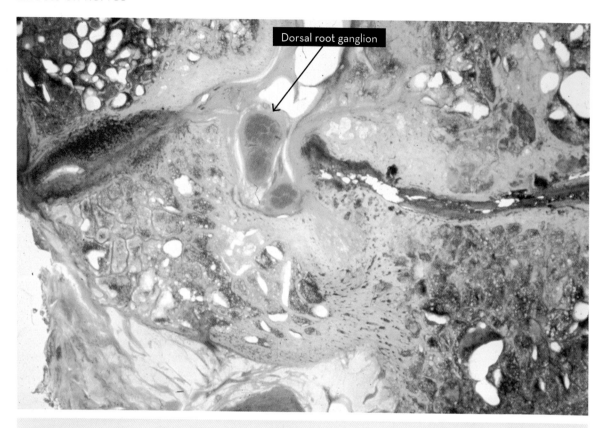

FIGURE 4.7A

A 100-micron stained coronal section of the C6–7 disc from an elderly subject.

This disc is completely resorbed and its lateral margin is encroaching on the intervertebral foramen. The nerve roots are flattened by the disc bulge.

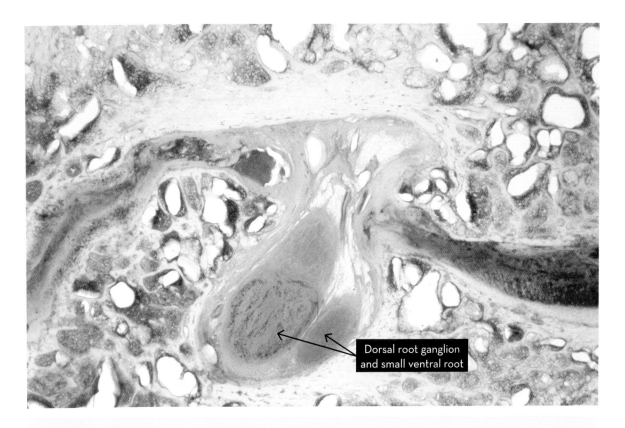

FIGURE 4.7B
A 100-micron stained coronal section of the C6–7 disc from another elderly subject.

This disc shows loss of disc height. Bony ridges at the lateral disc margins encroach on the intervertebral foramen, restricting the space for the nerve roots. The dorsal root ganglion lies above and lateral to the small motor root. The section also shows arthritic change in the facet joint with further encroachment on the foramen. The higher position and larger size of the dorsal root ganglion make it more vulnerable to pressure and distortion than the motor root with a greater likelihood of sensory effects.

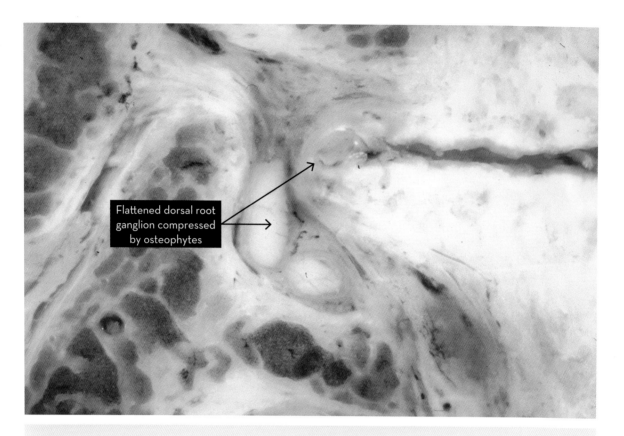

Flattened dorsal root ganglion compressed by osteophytes

FIGURE 4.8

A sagittal section showing osteophytes compressing and distorting a dorsal root ganglion.

A 2.5 mm thick unstained sagittal section of a lower cervical segment from an elderly subject shows the posterior part of a resorbed disc compressing the sensory nerve root. Disc resorption has left a very narrow empty space between the two sclerotic vertebrae. Large osteophytes project backwards from the vertebral margins, flattening the dorsal root ganglion in the intervertebral foramen. The facet joint also shows degenerative change with reduced articular cartilage and a large fatty inclusion.

Boyd-Clark and colleagues (2004) also reported degenerative changes with distortion and histological changes in the dorsal root ganglia.

Effects on vertebral arteries

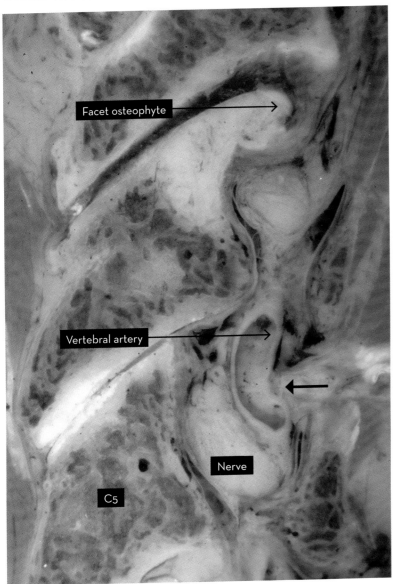

FIGURE 4.9
Effects on vertebral arteries.

Projection of disc and osteophytes in a 72-year-old man diverts the course of the vertebral artery, making it tortuous. Degenerative changes in discs and facets affect the vertebral artery, causing the originally straight artery to become tortuous (see thin arrow). This thick unstained sagittal section shows part of the artery being pushed outwards, curving around a white disc protrusion (see thick arrow). Above and below this level the artery would be held inwards by nerve roots and facet osteophytes. Note the degenerative changes in the upper facet joint: the joint is denuded of articular cartilage and a large sclerotic osteophyte projects forwards from the upper tip of the facet.

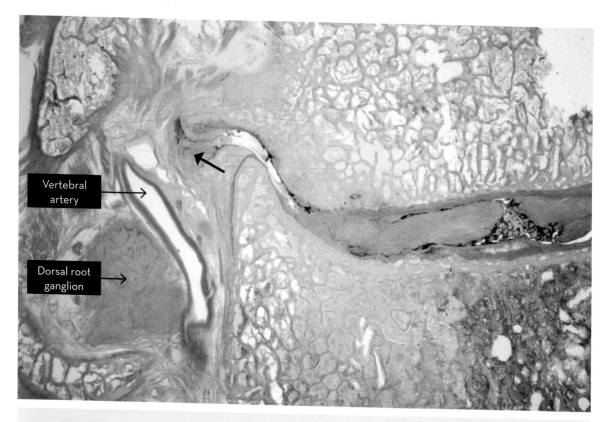

Vertebral artery

Dorsal root ganglion

FIGURE 4.10

Distortion of the vertebral artery by osteophytes in a 100-micron stained coronal section of the C5–6 disc from a 76-year-old man.

There is deviation of the vertebral artery from its original straight course, pushed laterally (see thick arrow) by uncovertebral osteophytes at the lateral margin of C5–6. The original outline of the uncus is visible with a lateral osteophytic accretion of new bone projecting laterally from the original outline. The osteophytes are capped by areas of cartilage which push the artery further laterally. The lower part of the artery is held medially by the dorsal root ganglion. Indian ink was injected into the central disc before processing to outline the fissures.

Effects on the spinal cord

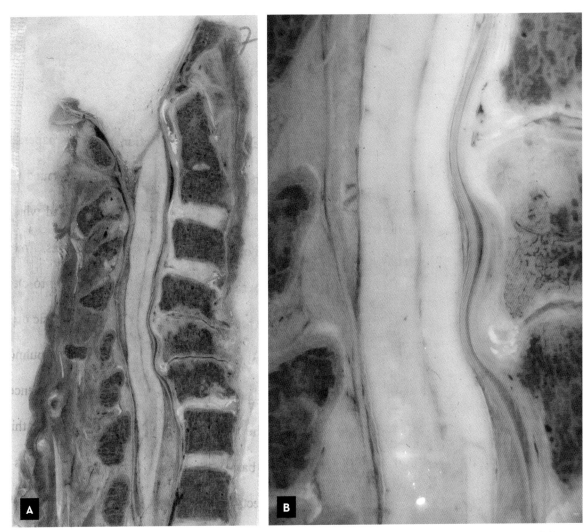

Figure 4.11A and B

Spinal stenosis due to disc degeneration.

This 2.5 mm thick midsagittal section is seen in low-power **(A)** and close-up **(B)**; it shows two 'hard' disc protrusions at C4–5 and C5–6 in a 72-year-old woman. The partly calcified protrusions indent the spinal cord. These indentations may occur without causing symptomatic myelopathy but they make the spinal cord more vulnerable to injury. If seen on MRI in a patient they require follow-up and may need surgical intervention if long tract signs begin to appear. In addition, multilevel degenerative changes have distorted the normal lordotic posture of the spine.

Other age changes

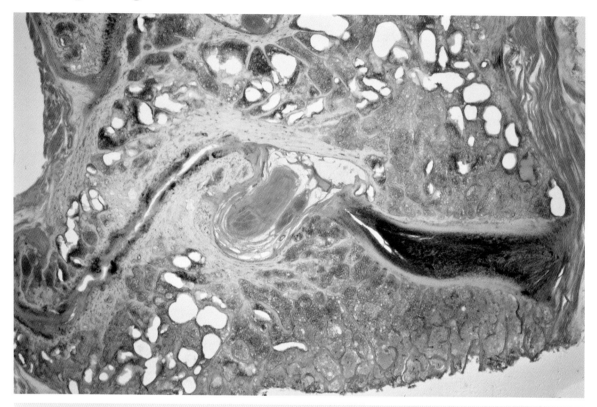

FIGURE 4.12A
Gross facet arthritic changes in an elderly subject (oblique section).

This lower cervical facet joint from an elderly subject shows advanced degenerative changes with loss of the articular cartilage and the presence of a facet osteophyte encroaching on the intervertebral foramen, compressing the nerve roots. Age changes in zygapophyseal facet joints generally occur at a later age than disc changes. The nerve root entrapment is principally due to facet arthritis.

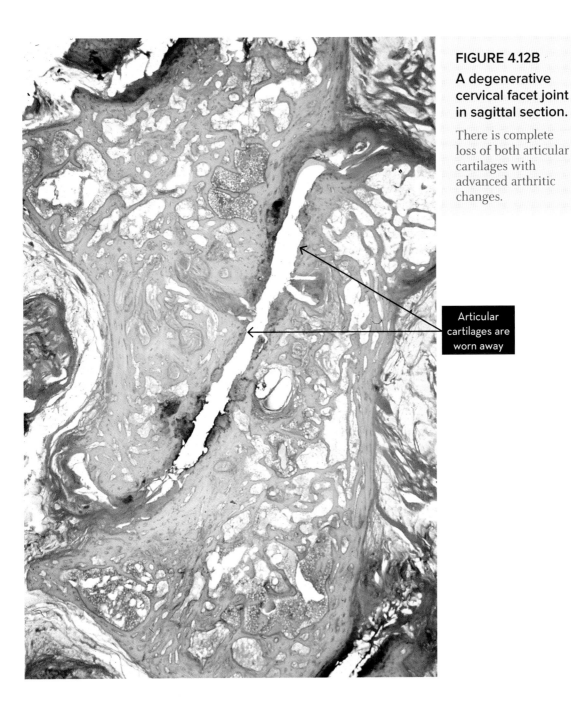

FIGURE 4.12B
A degenerative cervical facet joint in sagittal section.

There is complete loss of both articular cartilages with advanced arthritic changes.

Articular cartilages are worn away

Spontaneous interbody fusion in old age

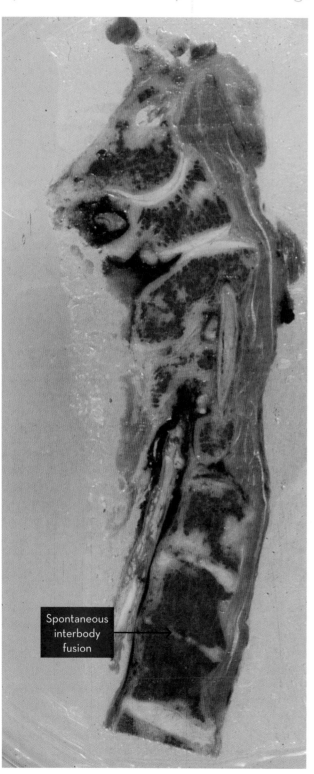

Spontaneous
interbody
fusion

FIGURE 4.13A

A sagittal section of spine from a 65-year-old man shows spontaneous interbody fusion, the end result of gross disc degeneration.

A laminectomy had been performed. The changes have distorted spinal posture causing torticollis, which made it impossible to section the whole spine in the same plane. Despite the gross subaxial degeneration the C0–1 and C1–2 joints are well preserved.

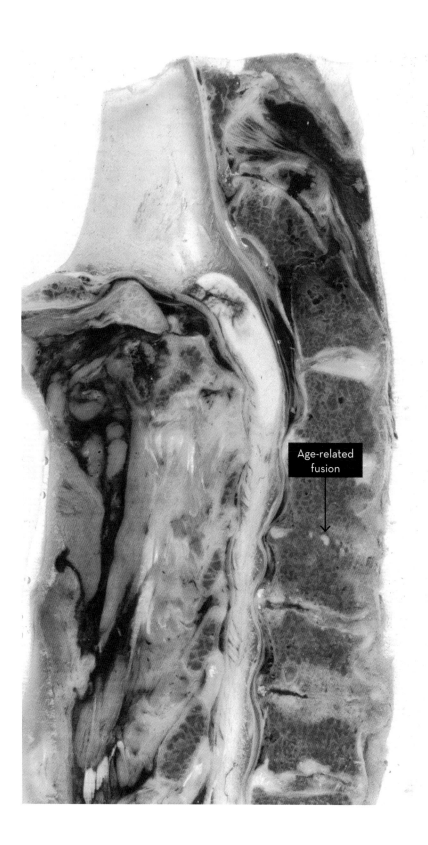

Age-related
fusion

FIGURE 4.13B
Spontaneous interbody fusion in an 86-year-old woman.

The stiff spine shows multilevel spinal canal stenosis and a high spinal cord injury with a dens fracture. The stiffness of the lower cervical spine made the upper level more vulnerable to injury, with a dens fracture and a high cord injury.

CHAPTER 5

BLUNT TRAUMA INJURIES TO THE CERVICAL SPINE

Blunt trauma tends to injure the most vulnerable parts of the cervical spine; it seeks out the weakest parts. The high frequency of injuries along the disc vertebral body junction suggests that this linear junction is weaker than the disc tissue itself, or the vertebral bone. Of the injuries along this junction, tears of the anterior annulus at its attachment to the vertebral rim are by far the most common.

DISC INJURIES

Rim lesions

The term 'rim lesion' was coined by Professor Barrie Vernon-Roberts of Adelaide to describe a split along the lumbar disc vertebral junction. These splits occur naturally in human lumbar discs but Vernon-Roberts and colleagues (1997) found that when they were surgically produced in sheep discs, they were precursors of disc degeneration. We found similar splits at the cervical disc vertebral junction at autopsy in subjects suffering blunt trauma. When seen on x-rays in living patients, these splits are called lucent clefts and they are attributed by radiologists to degenerative changes. However, in our study they are obviously a result of acute blunt trauma where there is bleeding into the annular tear from the vascular vertebral rim. Identical lesions (without bleeding) are common in chronic whiplash patients where there is a good case for regarding them as due to trauma.

The examples in Figure 5.1 are all from young adults who died from head injuries in motor vehicle accidents. The head impacts caused neck compression or extension. The lesions varied in size from localised anterior annular tears to small avulsions with more extensive disc vertebral separation (as in Figure 5.1B).

In our study we found that in blunt trauma deaths, anterior annular tears were by far the most common acute lesions in cervical spines. They were often multilevel injuries, most frequently at the upper junction of the annulus to the vertebral rim (see Figure 5.2). The lesions in Figures 5.1 and 5.2 were seen in midsagittal sections. Rim lesions or anterior annular tears occur in well-aligned spines with an intact anterior longitudinal ligament and often without visible injury to the longus colli muscles.

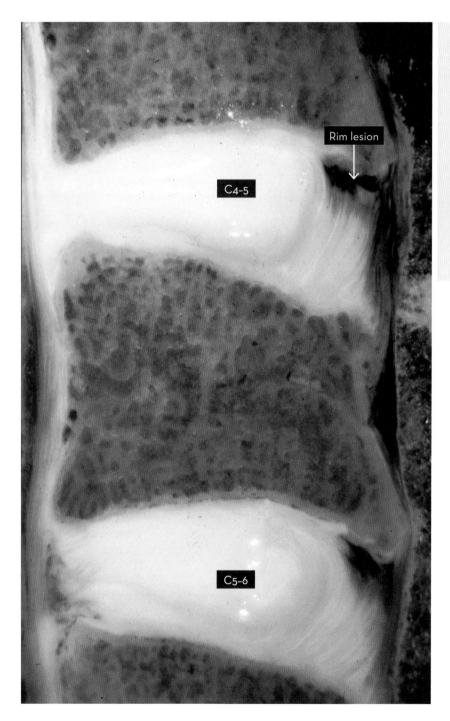

Rim lesion

C4-5

C5-6

FIGURE 5.1A
Anterior annular tears (rim lesions) in a thick sagittal section from a 20-year-old woman.

These acute lesions at the anterior vertebral rim are accompanied by local bleeding into the anterior annulus fibrosus, with spread of blood between the annular lamellae.

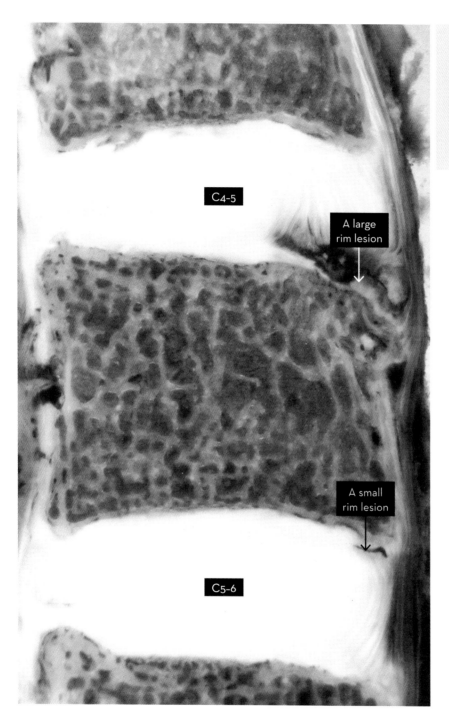

C4-5

A large
rim lesion

A small
rim lesion

C5-6

FIGURE 5.1B
More rim lesions in C4–5 and C5–6 due to blunt trauma in another young adult, as seen in sagittal section.

Figure 5.1 continues

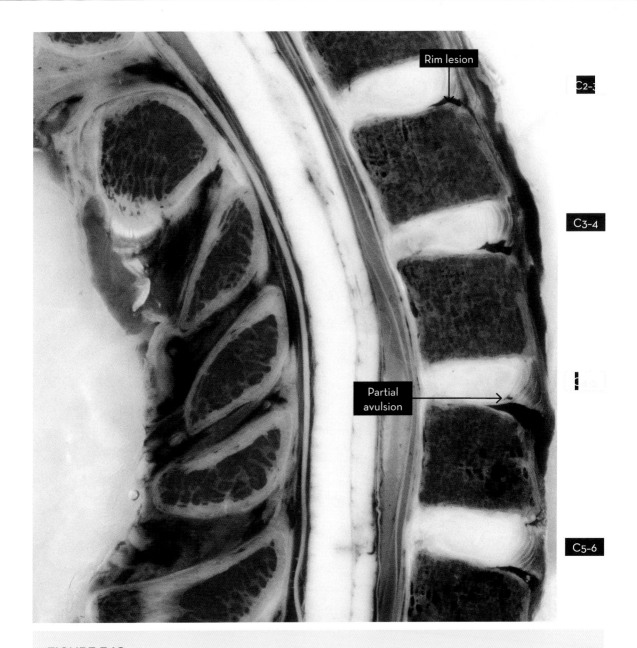

FIGURE 5.1C

Multilevel extension injuries in anterior discs seen in a midsagittal section from a young man.

These injuries are due to forced extension from anterior head impact in a motor vehicle accident. They vary from rim lesions to partial avulsion.

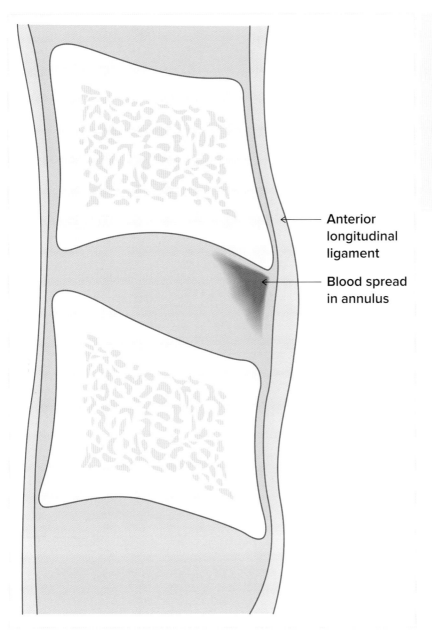

Anterior longitudinal ligament

Blood spread in annulus

FIGURE 5.2

Acute rim lesions show the spread of bleeding between the annular lamellae.

The longitudinal ligaments are intact. Rim lesions are often multilevel injuries.

Severe disc injuries

Avulsions

The most common severe disc injury in our study was linear avulsion of the disc along the disc vertebral junction.

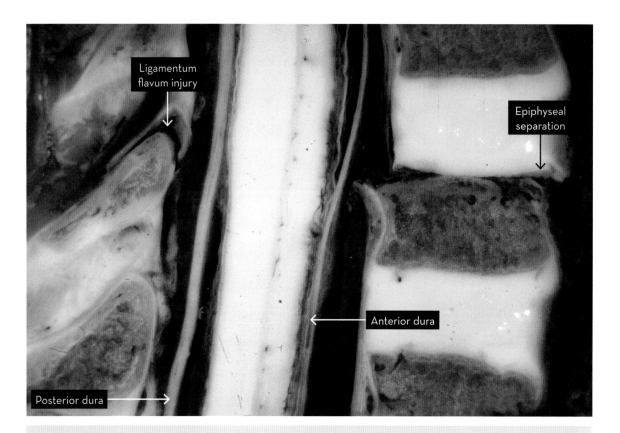

Ligamentum flavum injury

Epiphyseal separation

Anterior dura

Posterior dura

FIGURE 5.3
Epiphyseal separation in an infant seen in midsagittal section.

Avulsions tended to occur in young adults, but this 15-month-old infant shows a complete epiphyseal (cartilage plate) separation from the bony vertebral body resulting from an injury in a head-on collision. The spinal cord is intact but there is a separation of the ligamentum flavum from the lamina and there are extensive anterior and posterior epidural haematomas. The posterior dura is much thicker than the anterior dura (see Figure 2.13).

Our extensive studies of blunt trauma injuries to the cervical spine show that it is wrong to conclude that in extension trauma the most anterior structure will rupture first and then deeper structures will tear in series. A different capacity for stretch in different tissues is more important in determining the order of rupture. The short collagen fibres of the anterior annulus tear first, the much longer fibres of the anterior longitudinal ligament tear next and the compliant longus colli muscle fibres tear last.

Avulsions are diagnosed less often than herniations in clinical practice; they may be missed on imaging if intact anterior strap muscles remain capable of holding the structures together in a well-aligned spine.

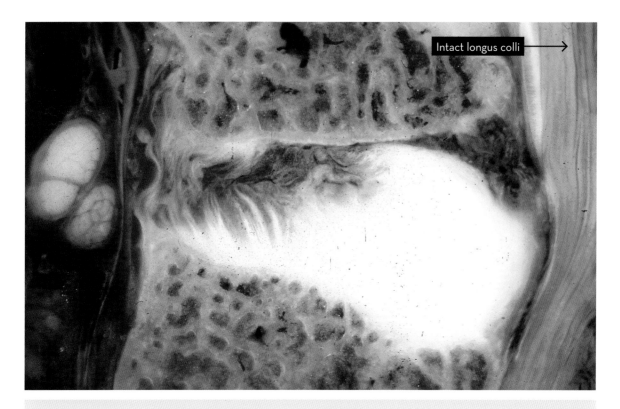

Intact longus colli

FIGURE 5.4A
Disc avulsion in a fatal car accident.

This 2.5 mm thick unstained sagittal section from a 42-year-old man shows a linear avulsion of two-thirds of the C6–7 disc from the vertebral body. The anterior longitudinal ligament is torn but the longus colli muscles on each side of the midline are intact. There is posterior disc bruising from axial compression and an epidural haematoma.

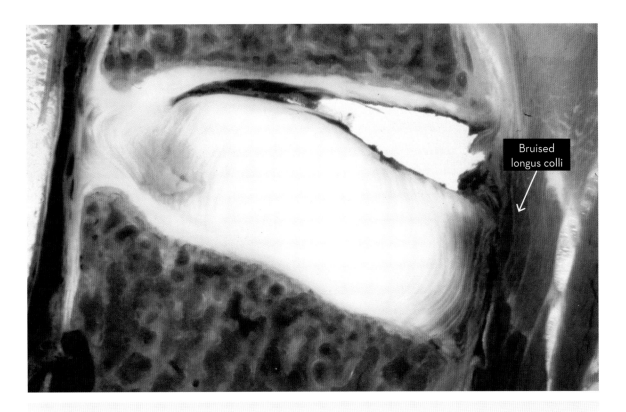

FIGURE 5.4B
Extensive disc avulsion.

This thick unstained parasagittal section shows an extensive linear avulsion of the C6–7 disc from the vertebral body in a 20-year-old man. The anterior longitudinal ligament is ruptured but the longus colli muscle, though bruised, is not ruptured.

Disc disruption

In subjects over 55 years of age with degenerative disc changes, clean-cut linear avulsions along the disc vertebral junction are unusual. Instead, we found irregular disc disruptions often accompanied by a 'tear-drop fracture' at the anterior margin of the vertebral body.

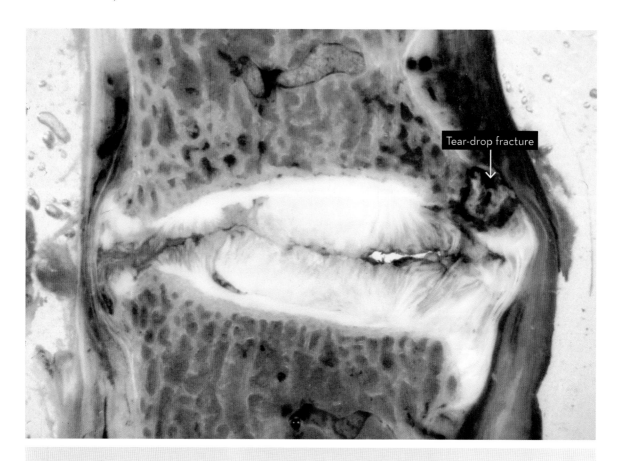

FIGURE 5.5A

Disc disruption shown in sagittal section.

In this 62-year-old man the age-related central fissure has extended into the anterior annulus of C5–6 and the lower anterior corner of the vertebral body above is fractured, with haemorrhage in the damaged longus colli muscle above the fracture.

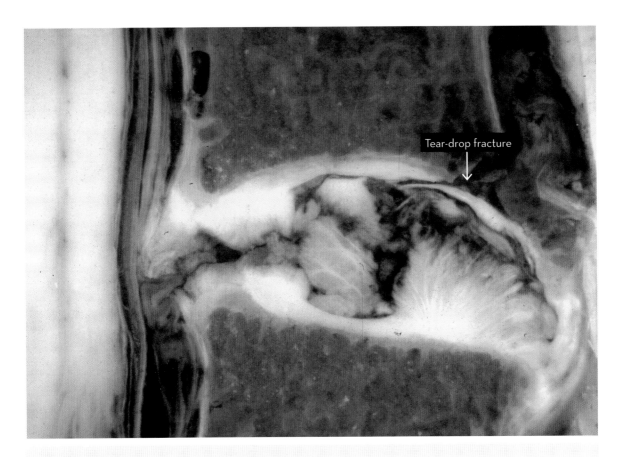

FIGURE 5.5B
Disc disruption shown in sagittal section.

In this 58-year-old man there is extensive disruption of a lower cervical disc with posterior disc herniation and an anterior tear-drop fracture above the disc.

Disc herniations

Disc herniations are the most common disc injury diagnosed clinically in moderate to severe blunt trauma.

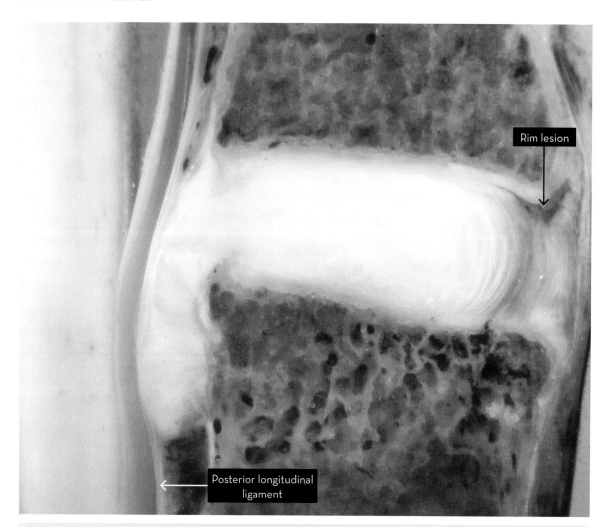

FIGURE 5.6A

Disc herniations.

A sagittal section of C6–7 from a 52-year-old man shows a posterior disc hernia that has migrated down behind the vertebral body below. The posterior longitudinal ligament is tented backwards close to the anterior dura and the cord. There is a rim lesion anteriorly with bleeding between the lamellae of the anterior annulus. There is a small area of bone bruising in the vertebral body directly below the rim lesion.

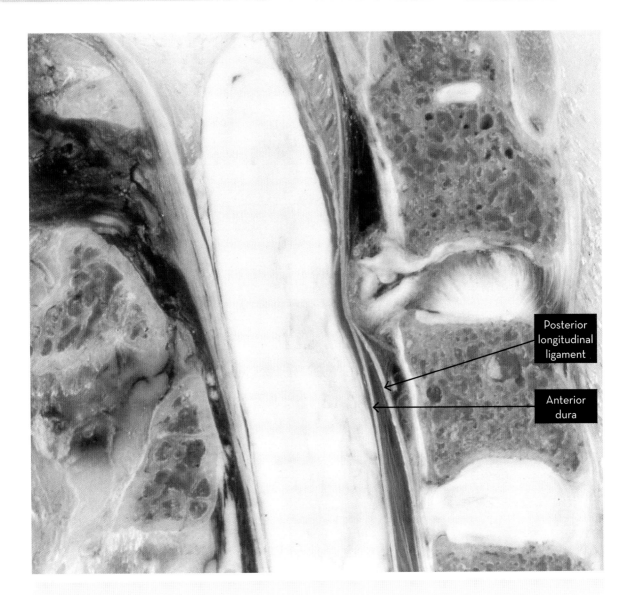

Posterior longitudinal ligament

Anterior dura

FIGURE 5.6B
Disc herniations.

This midline sagittal section of C2–3 is from a 22-year-old woman killed in a head-on collision causing anterior head impact and a neck extension injury. The disc hernia is large enough to indent the spinal cord. There is also damage to the ligamentum flavum with a posterior epidural haematoma. The disc hernia tents the posterior longitudinal ligament back without tearing it and allows dilation of the veins above and below the hernia.

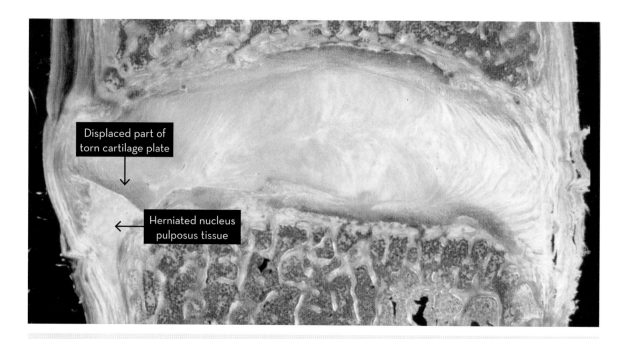

Displaced part of
torn cartilage plate

Herniated nucleus
pulposus tissue

FIGURE 5.7

An atypical posterior herniation in a 100-micron unstained sagittal section of C4–5 in a 32-year-old man injured in a car accident.

Part of the lower cartilage plate has been torn away from its normal position and displaced to the posterior disc margin leaving a step-like defect in the cartilage plate. Central disc material (white) has prolapsed beyond the displaced cartilage plate into the torn lower posterior annulus. (Dark ground illumination makes the cartilage plate appear blue.)

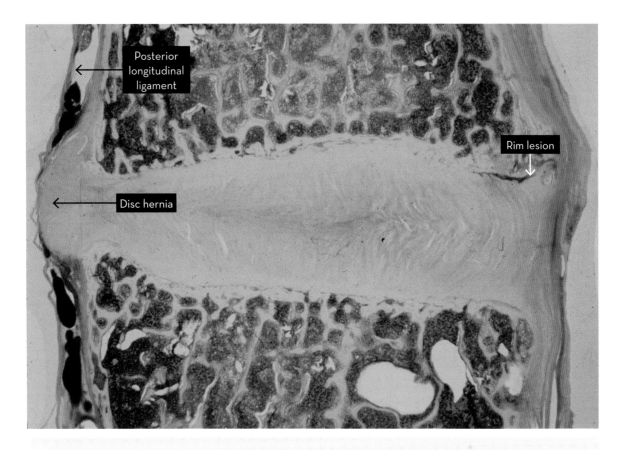

FIGURE 5.8

A 100-micron stained sagittal section of C6–7 shows a typical mushroom-shaped posterior disc herniation.

This disc is from a 32-year-old man killed in a car accident. The hernia has tented the posterior longitudinal ligament so that the veins above and below are dilated. There is also a small blood-filled rim lesion in the upper anterior annulus (rim lesions often accompany herniations).

Segmental frequency of major and minor disc lesions

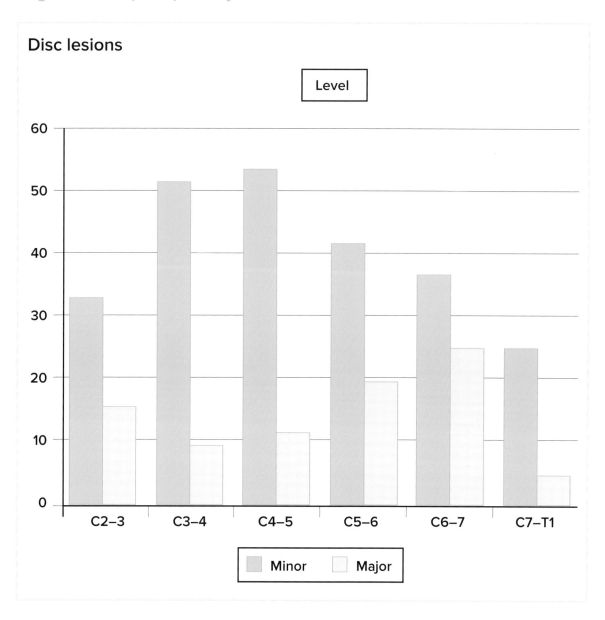

Figure 5.9

Segmental frequency of major and minor disc lesions.

Major disc injuries—avulsions, disruptions and herniations, shown in the light-green columns—are most common at C5–6 and C6–7, but rim lesions—shown in the dark-green columns—are most frequent at C3–4 and C4–5, where the facet angles are closer to the horizontal plane. This favours greater translation with shearing in the C3–4 and C4–5 discs on movement at these levels. In a measurement study of facet angles we found a strong correlation between more nearly horizontal facet angles and the presence of rim lesions. This suggests that rim lesions are due to shear injury in translation.

Disc injuries have been described by other authors (see, for example, Taylor, 2003; Jonsson et al., 1991; and Pettersson et al., 1997).

Traumatic disc herniations are well-known clinically but the high frequency of linear separation of the disc from the vertebral body in young adults, as found at autopsy in fatal blunt trauma, does not seem to be recognised in clinical practice. The importance of rim lesions as possible precursors of extensive disc degeneration in the cervical spine following whiplash injury appears to have been overlooked.

FACET INJURIES FROM BLUNT TRAUMA

Minor facet injuries from blunt trauma in young adults

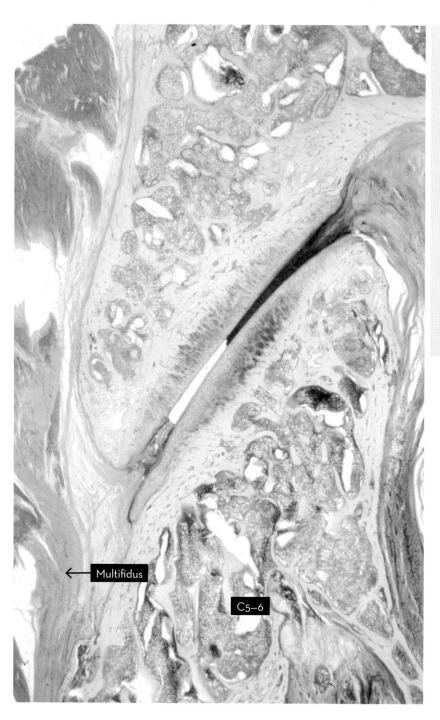

Multifidus

C5–6

FIGURE 5.10A

A bruised synovial fold with no articular cartilage or capsular damage in a 35-year-old man, shown in sagittal section.

Blunt trauma injuries to facet joints vary from simple synovial fold bruises to facet fractures.

The triangular synovial fold, enclosed by the multifidus, in the inferior recess appears uninjured.

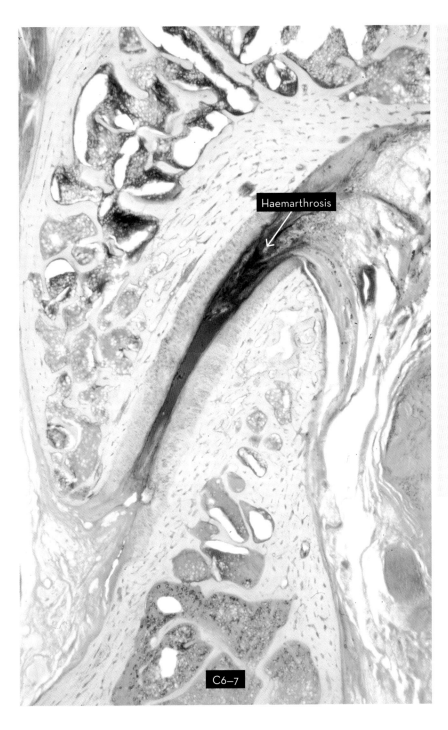

Haemarthrosis

C6–7

FIGURE 5.10B
Facet joint haemarthrosis shown in sagittal section.

A haemarthrosis is shown with blood right through the C6–7 joint from a ruptured synovial fold in a 35-year-old man. The vascular synovial folds move freely in and out of the joints in normal movement but the high-speed movement in a car accident can nip and bruise them. The joints are innervated by segmental medial branches of dorsal rami. These acute minor injuries would be painful but would probably heal quickly in survivors.

Articular cartilage injuries

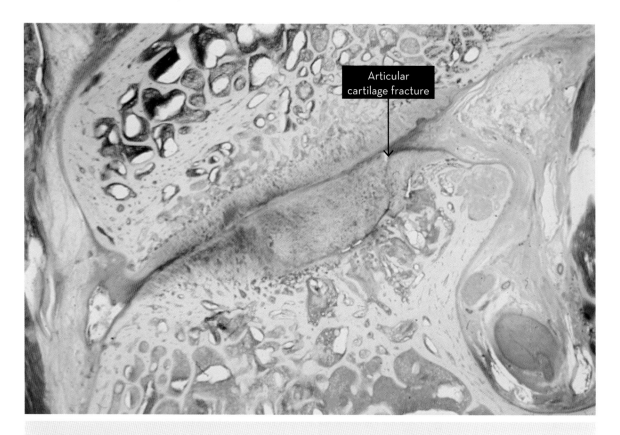

Articular
cartilage fracture

FIGURE 5.11A
Large loading forces in extension may injure the articular cartilage.

A 100-micron stained sagittal section shows a C3–4 facet from a 36-year-old man. There is a semi-circular fracture of the articular cartilage sustained in fatal motor vehicle accident due to extension compression.

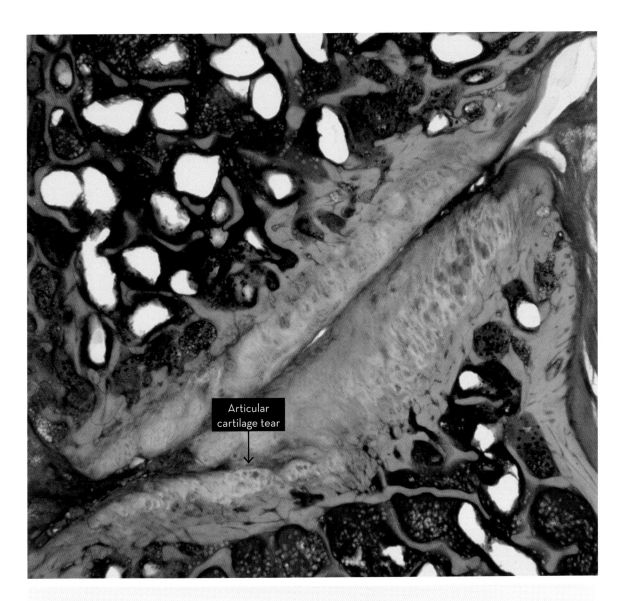

Articular cartilage tear

FIGURE 5.11B

A sagittal section of the C3–4 joint from a 36-year-old man showing a cartilage tear due to severe blunt trauma.

Injuries to avascular tissues do not heal readily so severe cartilage injuries would be likely to lead to early-onset osteoarthritis in survivors.

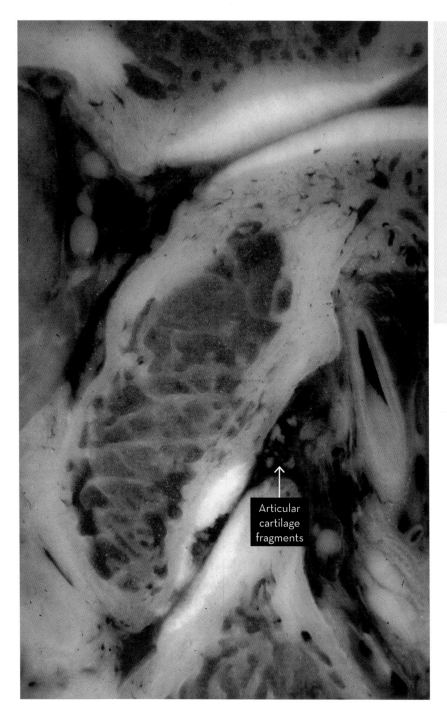

Articular
cartilage
fragments

FIGURE 5.12A
A C2–3 facet injury shown in a thick sagittal section.

This flexion injury at C2–3 in a 28-year-old man resulted from hyperflexion when the sharp tip of the lower facet 'dug out' fragments of articular cartilage from the upper facet; the detached cartilage fragments are seen in the upper anterior joint recess.

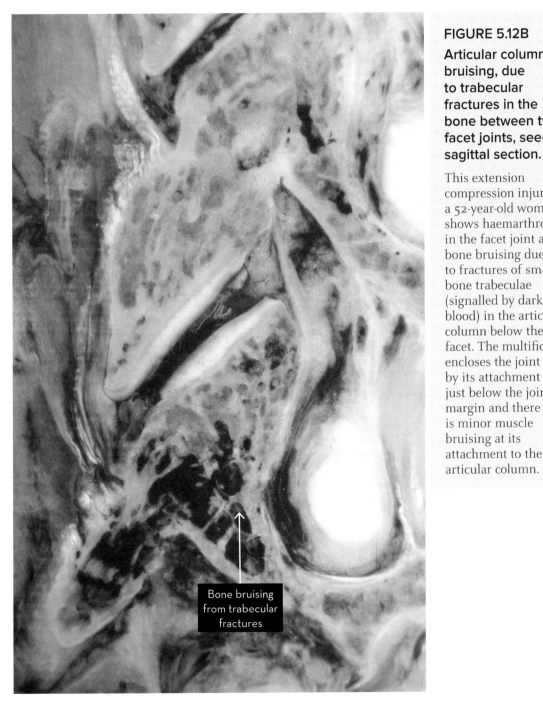

Bone bruising
from trabecular
fractures

FIGURE 5.12B
Articular column bruising, due to trabecular fractures in the bone between two facet joints, seen in sagittal section.

This extension compression injury in a 52-year-old woman shows haemarthrosis in the facet joint and bone bruising due to fractures of small bone trabeculae (signalled by dark blood) in the articular column below the facet. The multifidus encloses the joint by its attachment just below the joint margin and there is minor muscle bruising at its attachment to the articular column.

Facet fractures

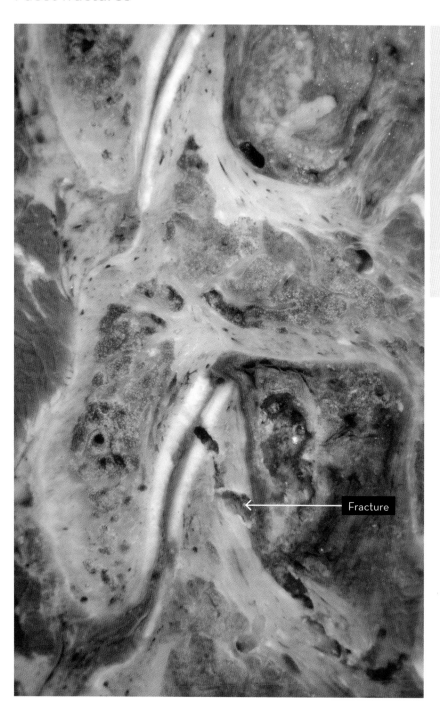

Fracture

FIGURE 5.13A
Facet fracture shown in sagittal section.

This facet tip fracture at C7–T1 in a young man was caused by a blow to the top of the head. He suffered cord concussion and death from asphyxia. There was a similar injury at C6–7 and he also showed bruising of several discs.

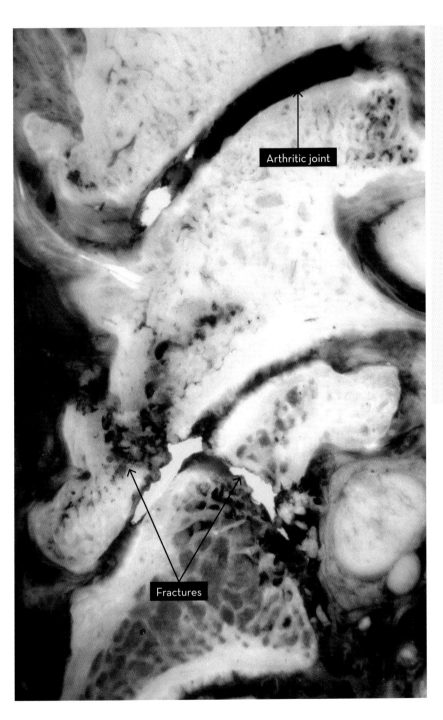

FIGURE 5.13B
Facet fractures shown in sagittal section.

These facet fractures in a 56-year-old man were caused in a roll-over accident with death from 'multiple injuries'. The lower end of C6 and the upper end of C7 are fractured, with extensive bleeding into the muscles behind the C6–7 facet. There is haemarthrosis in C5–6 which, like C4–5, is denuded of cartilage due to longstanding degenerative change.

Segmental frequency of major and minor facet injuries

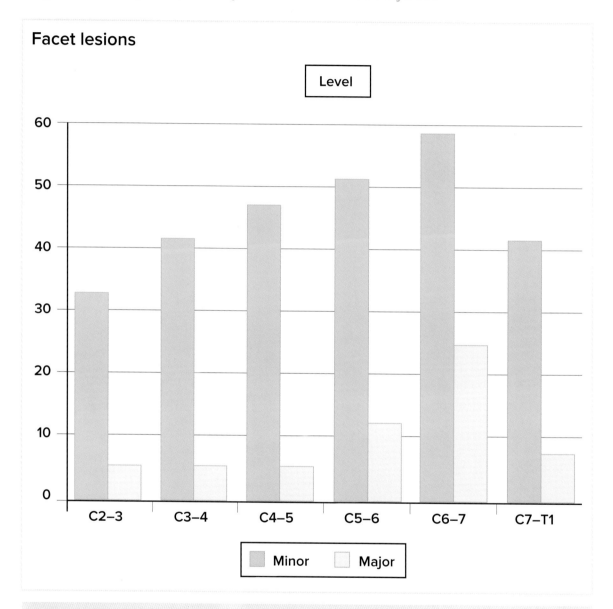

Figure 5.14

Segmental frequency of major and minor facet injuries.

The dark-green columns show the frequency of soft-tissue injuries and the light-green columns show the frequency of facet fractures. There is a progressive segmental increase in both soft-tissue injuries (including articular cartilage injuries) and facet fractures from C2–3 down to C6–7. The most mobile segments at C5–6 and C6–7 show the highest frequency of both types of injury. The high frequency of severe disc injuries and facet fractures at C5–6 and C6–7 correlates with the frequency of spinal cord injury at the same levels in patients admitted to spinal injury units.

CHAPTER 6

SPINAL CORD AND DORSAL ROOT GANGLION INJURIES

In our study, 55% of injuries seen in autopsy showed fracture dislocations but this chapter does not deal in detail with fracture dislocations and spinal cord injuries as these are well described in orthopaedic and neurosurgery texts. Lower cervical spinal cord injuries causing quadriplegia are generally managed in specialist spinal injury units. High cervical fracture dislocations with fatal high cord or lower brainstem injuries are of more interest to forensic pathologists than to clinicians. Here we deal mainly with injuries in well-aligned spines because patients with these injuries are more likely to survive to be seen by clinicians.

SPINAL CORD INJURIES

High spinal cord injuries

Figure 6.1 shows two examples of high spinal cord injuries that illustrate the predisposition to high injuries in subjects with stiff lower cervical spines.

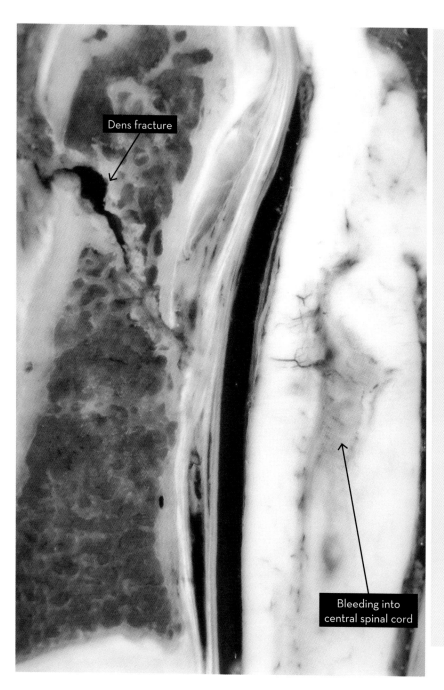

Dens fracture

Bleeding into
central spinal cord

FIGURE 6.1A
A midsagittal section showing a high spinal cord injury.

A dens fracture with spinal cord injury in an 86-year-old woman, resulting from a simple fall with anterior head impact. There is central haemorrhage in the cord opposite the dens fracture. The subaxial spine was stiff due to multiple interbody fusions. This is one of three cases in our study of high spinal cord injury in elderly subjects who suffered a fall with a head impact. The frail elderly are vulnerable to trauma from falls. Dens fractures are the most common upper cervical fractures.

In a survey of 21,672 premature deaths in nursing homes Ibrahim and colleagues (2017) found falls to be one of the most common causes of death.

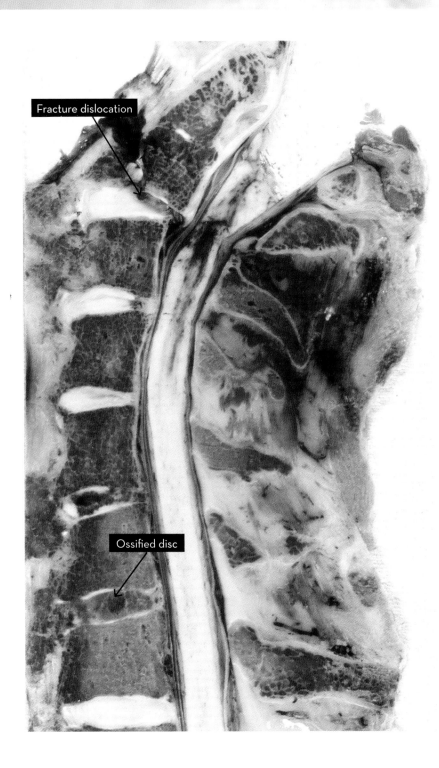

Fracture dislocation

Ossified disc

FIGURE 6.1B
A sagittal section showing a high spinal cord injury.

The spine from a middle-aged man with ankylosing spondylitis shows disc ossification and interbody fusions with a continuous bar of bone splinting the front of the column. His fatal car accident was at low speed and he suffered an anterior head impact, causing an extension injury with C2–3 fracture dislocation and extensive cord injury with central cord bleeding.

High central cord injuries

Spinal cord injuries above C4 paralyse respiration and result in death from asphyxia. Cord injuries in the lower cervical spine cause quadriplegia with loss of distal upper limb function, paralysis of lower limbs and loss of bowel and bladder control.

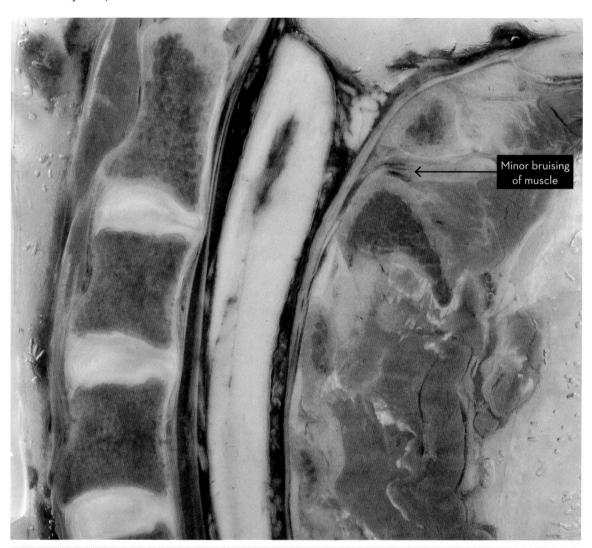

Minor bruising of muscle

FIGURE 6.2A

An example of high central cord injury in a midsagittal section.

This spine shows a small linear area of central haemorrhage at the C2 level in a 17-year-old woman from a hyperextension injury when her stationary vehicle was struck from behind. The spine remained well-aligned and apart from the cord injury there were only tiny haemorrhages into the high posterior spinal muscle between the C1 and C2 arches. It was assumed that marked hyperextension in a mobile young spine caused sudden severe narrowing of the spinal canal with cord trauma.

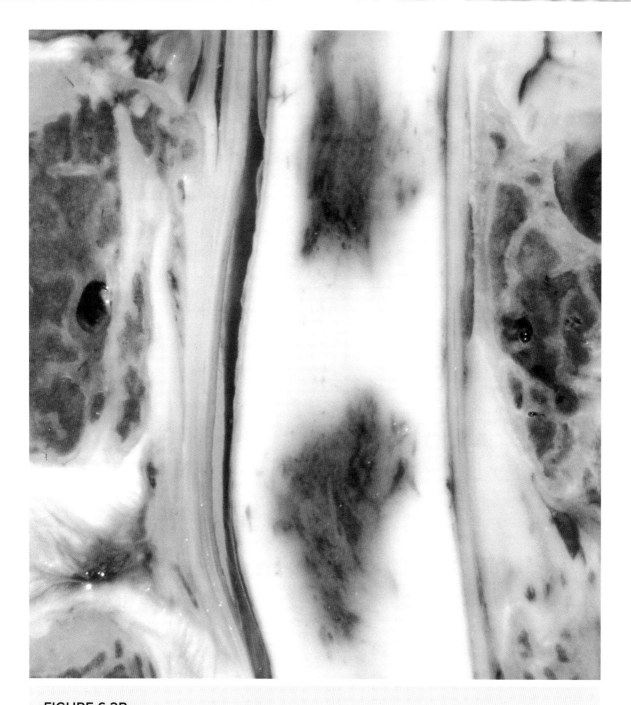

FIGURE 6.2B
High central cord injuries in midsagittal section.

These spinal cord injuries at the C3 and C4 levels are seen in a midsagittal section. They resulted from a surfing accident in a 62-year-old man. There were anterior disc avulsions at C3–4, C4–5 and C5–6. The spinal canal was already narrow and hyperextension would have compressed the upper cord.

DORSAL ROOT GANGLION INJURIES

In our study we found that dorsal root ganglion injuries were very common in well-aligned spines subject to blunt trauma. These were due to stretch injuries in extension or side bending.

The large oval cervical dorsal root ganglia contain the cell bodies of bipolar neurons (Figure 6.6) connecting peripheral sensory endings with the central nervous system. The ganglia contain many thin-walled blood vessels. They lie in the lateral parts of the intervertebral foramina where the lower cervical ganglia occupy a large percentage of the space between the uncus and the facet joint. Dorsal root ganglion injuries were the most common nervous system injuries in this study and damage to the small blood vessels in the ganglia made naked-eye recognition of injury possible.

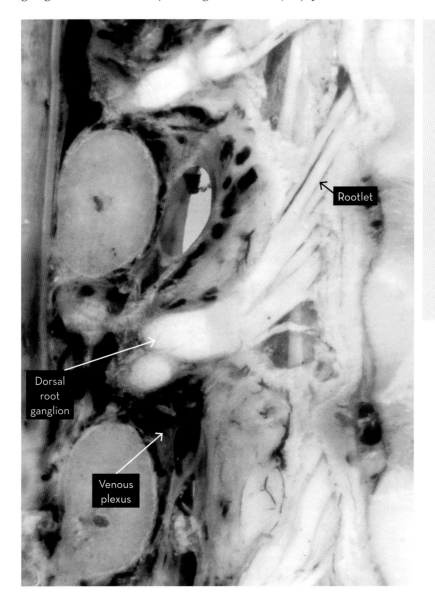

Rootlet

Dorsal root ganglion

Venous plexus

FIGURE 6.3A
Dorsal root ganglion vulnerability to injury.

A thick sagittal slice from an autopsy shows the anterolateral course of the dorsal nerve rootlets to the dorsal root ganglion. This oblique course makes them vulnerable to overstretch in both side bending and extension. In the lateral spinal canal a venous epidural plexus surrounds the nerve roots.

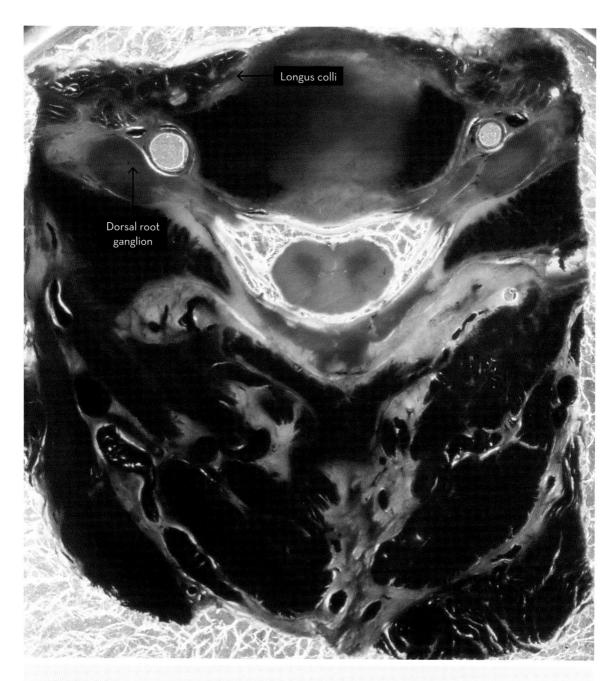

FIGURE 6.3B
Dorsal root ganglion vulnerability to injury.

This transverse section of the neck from a 72-year-old woman shows the gross difference between the large mass of posterior muscles and the much smaller anterior strap muscles, the longus colli. The small anterior muscles give scant protection against extension forces. The oval dorsal root ganglia lie in front of the articular columns behind the vertebral arteries. The dorsal roots pass forwards and laterally. (Compare with Figure 3.2.)

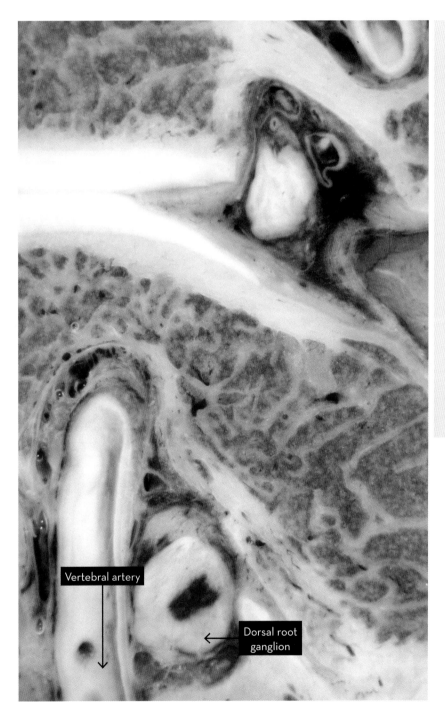

Vertebral artery

Dorsal root ganglion

FIGURE 6.4A
Central haemorrhage in dorsal root ganglia.

The right C3 dorsal root ganglion from a 17-year-old woman killed in a side impact motor vehicle accident is shown in sagittal section; there is bleeding into the central part of the ganglion.

The vertebral artery lies anterior to the ganglion and shows the origin of one of its segmental branches in the wall of the artery. Part of the C1–2 joint with the C2 dorsal root ganglion is seen above.

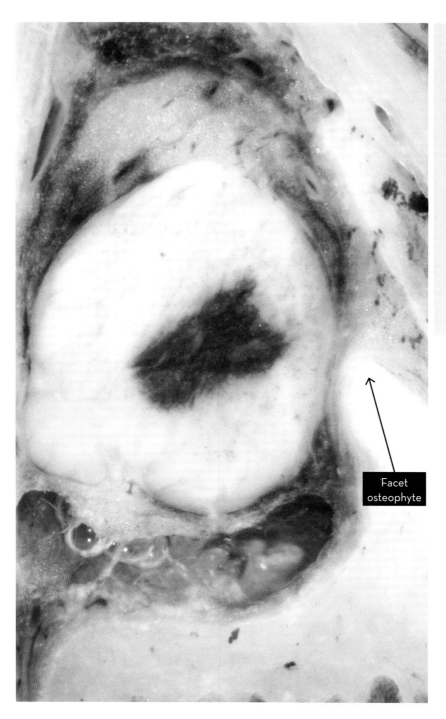

FIGURE 6.4B

Central haemorrhage in a dorsal root ganglion shown in sagittal section.

A closer view of the injured ganglion shows how closely it is related to the upper pole of the C2–3 facet joint.

The dorsal root ganglion injuries appeared to be stretch injuries in extension or side bending.

Facet osteophyte

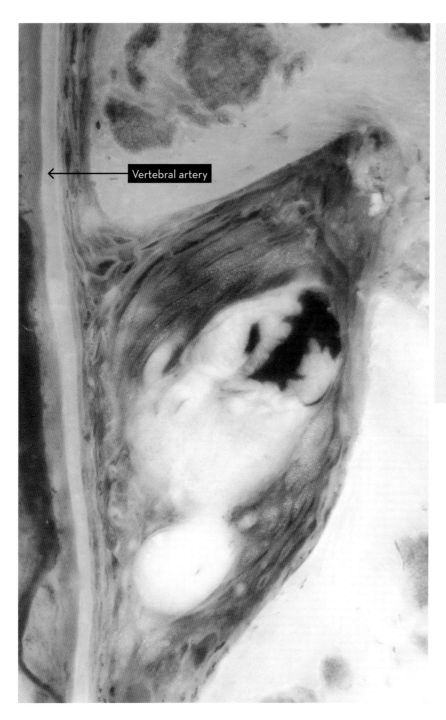

Vertebral artery

FIGURE 6.5A
Haemorrhage in a dorsal root ganglion shown in sagittal section.

A C6 dorsal root ganglion injury from a 33-year-old man who died from a 3-metre fall onto his head and shoulders. The ganglion shows interstitial haemorrhage. The nerve roots are enclosed in layered areolar tissue in the intervertebral foramen. The posterior wall of the vertebral artery is seen in front of the nerve roots.

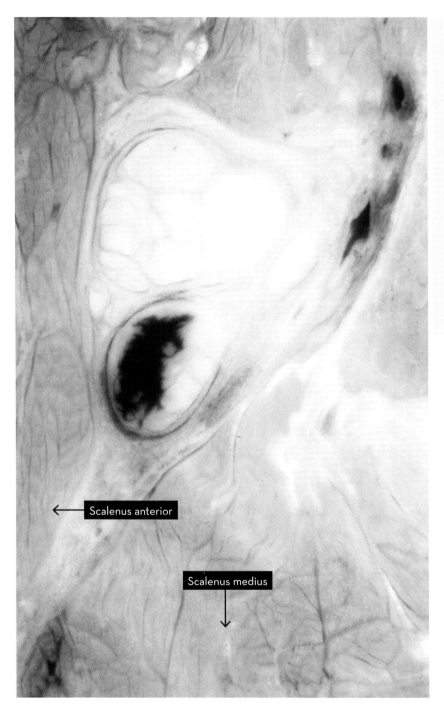

FIGURE 6.5B
Haemorrhage in a motor root shown in sagittal section.

This shows our only case of haemorrhage into the motor root—all other haemorrhages were into the sensory dorsal root ganglion. The nerve roots emerge from the intervertebral foramen to lie between the scalenus medius and the scalenus anterior.

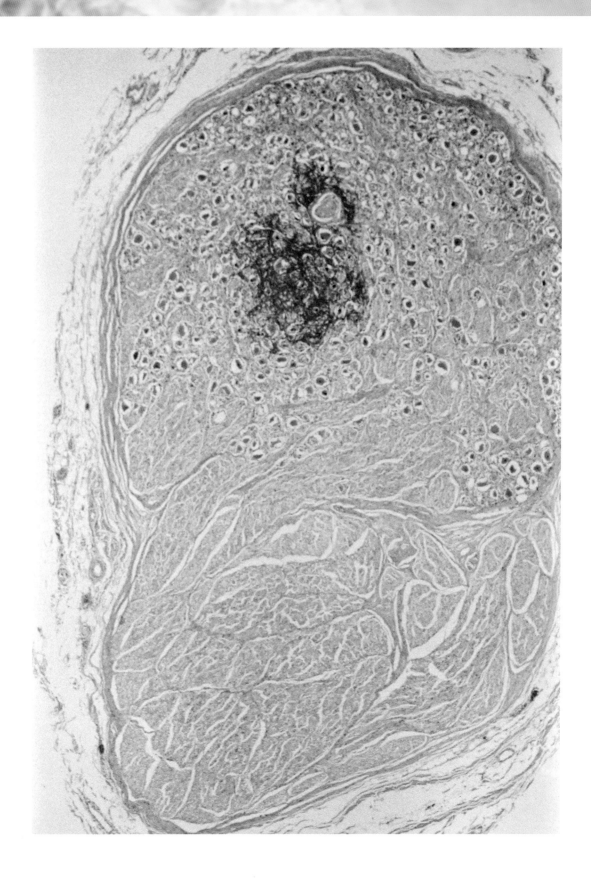

FIGURE 6.6

Haemorrhage seen in a thin section.

The dark dots in the upper part of the dorsal root ganglion indicate the cell bodies of bipolar sensory neurons which connect peripheral sensory endings with the spinal cord.

Microscopic examination of thin sections of injured dorsal root ganglia confirmed the presence of central haemorrhage due to rupture of the thin-walled vessels that traverse each ganglion. Dorsal root ganglion haemorrhage was found in 13.8% of the 109 individuals in the early part of the study. Notably it was found more often in individuals who survived the injury for more than 2 hours. Short-term survival allowed time for haemorrhage into the ganglion, as a marker of acute injury. Most dorsal root ganglion injuries were accompanied by minor musculoskeletal injuries from motor vehicle accidents, although a few ganglion injuries were found in 'shaken babies'. C5 and C8 at the upper and lower ends of the brachial plexus were the most commonly injured ganglia. Microscopy of injured ganglia in thin sections found axonal disruption accompanying haemorrhage in 6 of the 15 ganglia examined.

The frequency of cervical dorsal root ganglion injury in blunt trauma

In those who survived injury between 2 hours and 7 days the percentage showing haemorrhage into the dorsal root ganglion was 34.5%. In the 9 people who survived for longer than a week no dorsal root ganglion haemorrhage was found (see Table 6.1) and it is possible that any acute bleeding into the dorsal root ganglia had been resorbed.

TABLE 6.1	Effect of survival time on the prevalence of dorsal root ganglion injury found in 109 cases of blunt trauma			
	Survival time			
	<1.5 hours	**2–24 hours**	**2–7 days**	**8–90 days**
Number of deaths from blunt trauma	71	16	13	9
Number with dorsal root ganglion haemorrhage	5	7	3	0
Percentage with dorsal root ganglion haemorrhage	7.0%	43.8%	23.1%	0

Most dorsal root ganglion injuries were seen in individuals with relatively minor cervical spinal injuries, suggesting that it is not necessary to sustain very severe forms of blunt trauma to injure the dorsal root ganglion. These injuries were seen in 'shaken babies', in adults who died from a fall onto the head and shoulders, and most often in motor vehicle accidents, with especially severe bleeding from side impacts.

The possibility of dorsal root ganglion injuries should be considered in chronic whiplash-associated disorder with neuropathic pain. Dorsal root ganglion injuries, especially when there is axonal damage as well as haemorrhage in the ganglia, may account for the neuropathic pain often seen in patients with chronic whiplash-associated disorder. Some patients with severe neuropathic pain even present with an arm in a sling as it is 'too painful to move' and examination finds a strongly positive brachial plexus stretch test. As well as somatic neurological symptoms there are often autonomic sympathetic reactive symptoms. Quintner (1989) found that 55 of 61 patients with arm pain and paraesthesia showed signs of hypersensitive neural tissues with a positive brachial plexus test. In a review of the evidence for whiplash injuries, James Elliott (2011) noted that 25% of whiplash patients had radicular symptoms combined with disc injuries. Further data can be found in Taylor, Twomey and Kakulas (1998). Other published work supports the presence of nerve root injuries in whiplash (see Ide, Ide & Yamaga, 2001; Ortongren et al., 1996; Svensson et al., 1998; Guez et al., 2003; Tominaga, Ivancic & Panjabi, 2006; Waxman & Rizzo, 1996).

CHAPTER 7

INJURIES TO OTHER TISSUES

So far this study has concentrated on injuries to the cervical joints and nerves but we also noted injuries to other tissues, including injuries to the ligamentum flavum (Figure 7.1), muscles (Figures 7.2 and 7.3) and vertebral arteries (Figures 7.4 and 7.5).

TEARS OF THE LIGAMENTUM FLAVUM

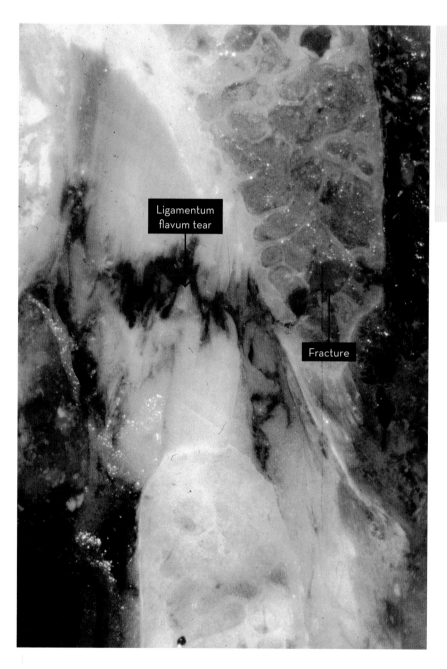

Ligamentum
flavum tear

Fracture

FIGURE 7.1A
Tear of the ligamentum flavum shown in sagittal section.

The ligamentum flavum has torn away from the lamina, breaking off a small part of the lamina.

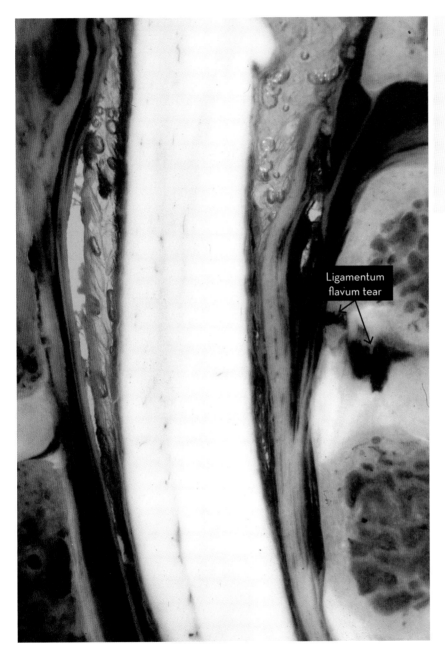

Ligamentum
flavum tear

FIGURE 7.1B

Tear of the ligamentum flavum shown in sagittal section.

The ligamentum flavum has torn away from the lamina, breaking off a tiny part of the lamina.

Injuries to the alar and transverse ligaments have also been described in MRI studies but the sagittal sections in this study do not reveal these injuries (see Vetti et al., 2011).

MUSCLE INJURIES

Muscle injuries are not a major theme in this atlas. Bleeding into muscles was a common finding in our study, but it was often due to injuries to underlying bones or joints. There is a growing body of literature describing reactive muscle changes in chronic whiplash-associated disorder, including pseudohypertrophy, atrophy and dysfunction (see, for example, Scott, Jull & Sterling, 2005; and Jull, Kristiansson & Dall'Alba, 2004). Chronic muscle dysfunction may be a reaction to chronic pain in the associated joints. In whiplash-associated disorder, tenderness from an enthesopathy may be difficult to distinguish from joint tenderness.

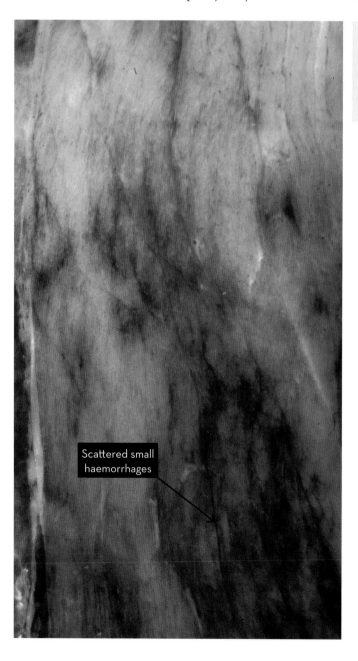

Scattered small haemorrhages

FIGURE 7.2A
Bleeding into muscles.

Multiple small muscle tears with haemorrhages.

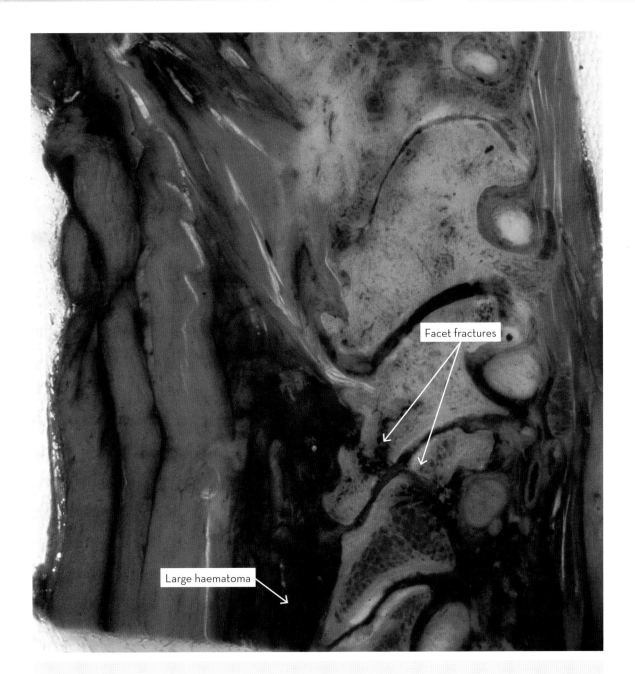

FIGURE 7.2B
Bleeding into muscles shown in sagittal section.

Intramuscular haematoma from injury to underlying bones in a 57-year-old woman. There are also gross degenerative changes in the facet joints above the injury with complete loss of articular cartilage at C6–7.

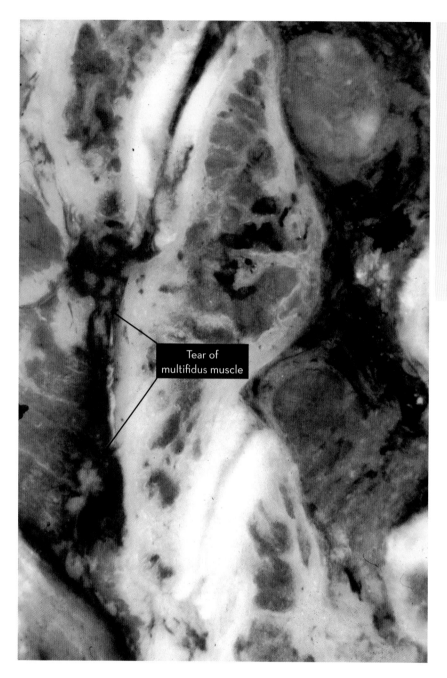

Tear of
multifidus muscle

FIGURE 7.3A
Muscle injuries shown in sagittal section. These injuries often occur at their areas of attachment to bone—their entheses.

A major tear of the multifidus muscle off its attachment to the articular column at C7 in a 57-year-old woman.

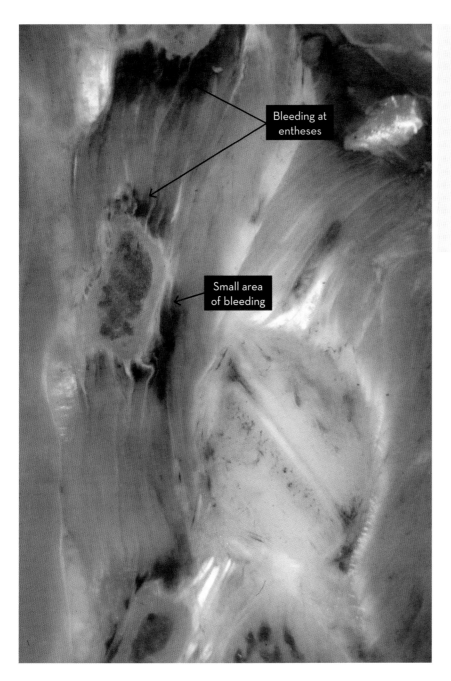

Bleeding at
entheses

Small area
of bleeding

FIGURE 7.3B
Muscle injuries shown in sagittal section at their areas of attachment to bone.

Multiple small localised areas of bleeding due to muscle injuries at their points of attachment.

VERTEBRAL ARTERY INJURIES

Vertebral artery damage most often accompanies fracture dislocations. It was not common in injured, well-aligned spines but three examples from well-aligned spines are illustrated in Figures 7.4 and 7.5. According to Vanessis (1987), most vertebral artery injuries are above the foramen magnum where the artery pierces the dura. The vertebral arteries supply the hindbrain and the upper spinal cord. Unilateral damage to a vertebral artery in a survivor may have less effect than expected, since the two vertebral arteries communicate intracranially with each other and with both internal carotid arteries in the circle of Willis. Vertebral artery asymmetry is common and the effect of a vertebral artery injury would tend to be more severe when the larger of the two asymmetrical arteries is injured.

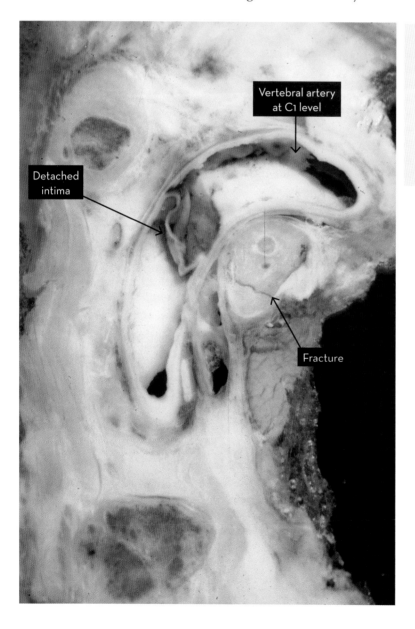

Vertebral artery
at C1 level

Detached
intima

Fracture

FIGURE 7.4A
Vertebral artery injury.

A sagittal section shows vertebral artery traumatic intimal dissection at the C1 level with a small associated undisplaced fracture of the posterior arch of C1.

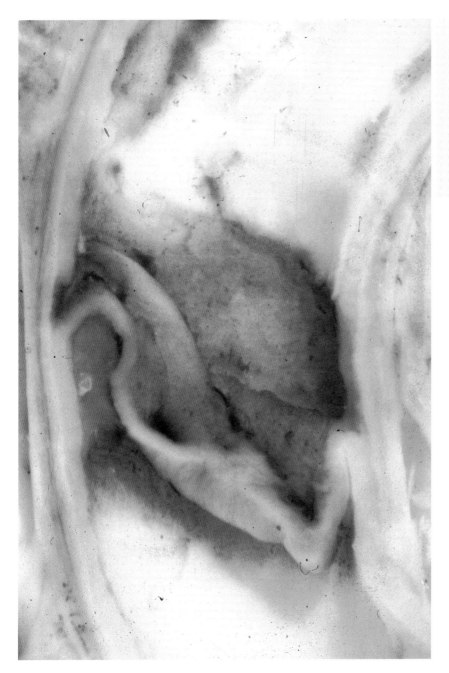

FIGURE 7.4B
Vertebral artery injury shown in sagittal section.

A closer view of the reflected flap of intima.

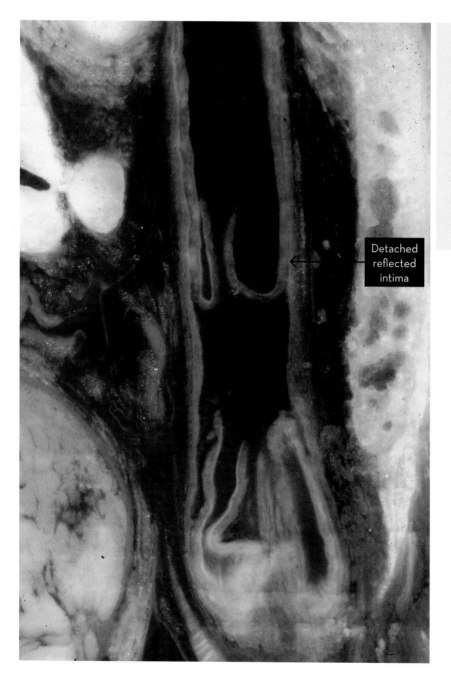

Detached reflected intima

FIGURE 7.5A
Vertebral artery dissection in the lower cervical spine.

A further example of intimal dissection in sagittal section. The direction of blood flow has flapped the dissected intima upwards.

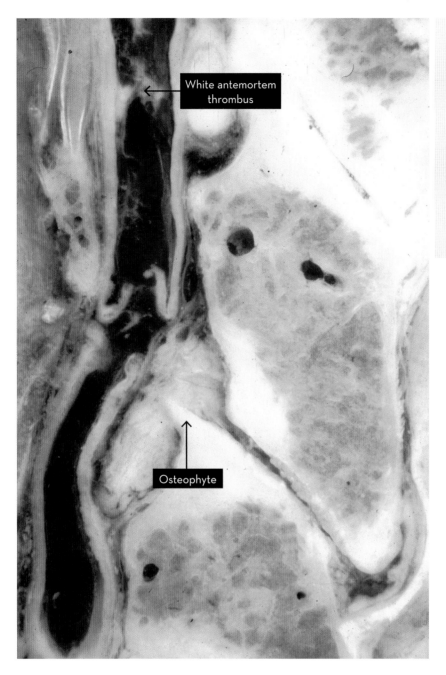

White antemortem thrombus

Osteophyte

FIGURE 7.5B
Vertebral artery dissection at C6.

The dissection has been provoked by the impingement of a sharp facet osteophyte on the artery wall. There is an antemortem thrombus (white) in the clot above the dissection.

CHAPTER 8

WHIPLASH INJURIES

Chapters 5, 6 and 7 describe acute blunt trauma injuries. This chapter examines persisting whiplash injuries in patients with chronic whiplash-associated disorder (WAD) and their relevance to chronic nociceptive pain arising in the injured structures.

The presence and identification of traumatic lesions in whiplash patients to account for their pain has been a matter of controversy. Bogduk's group in Newcastle (NSW) showed that they could reliably identify a painful facet, but they did not demonstrate the hypothetical lesions presumed to be responsible for the pain (Barnsley, Lord & Bogduk, 1994; Lord et al., 1996). Subsequent reviews support their conclusions (Engel et al., 2016; Persson et al., 2016; Smith et al., 2014; Smith et al., 2016).

In autopsy studies, plain x-rays at postmortem failed to demonstrate most soft-tissue whiplash lesions (Jonsson et al., 1991; Taylor & Twomey, 2005). Jonsson and colleagues (1991) found in a study of 22 road trauma deaths that 198 lesions found at autopsy were missed on postmortem x-rays. In a later study of 50 whiplash patients Jonsson and colleagues (1994) found at MRI that 10 patients had large disc herniations; at surgery they also found that MRI had underestimated the severity of the disc injuries. While MRI and CT scans are capable of demonstrating disc herniations, these investigations are often completed when the acute pain has failed to resolve and when signs of acute injury such as local haemorrhage may be resorbed.

In this chapter we demonstrate at autopsy persisting or altered whiplash lesions found 1–5 years after the initial injury when the patients died of some other cause and compare them with lesions found in living patients. The six case reports illustrated come from autopsies of survivors of whiplash injury who later died from other causes. The availability of clinical information of the signs and symptoms in these cases varied widely from the extensive information, including specialist reviews, provided in Case 1 to the paucity of clinical information of symptoms and signs in Case 4, where we relied on a brief report of the history of injury and chronic pain. We describe these lesions and, where possible, relate them to the history of the distribution of chronic pain in those who died and came to autopsy. Our main objective has been to find lesions at autopsy that can be attributable to the previous whiplash injury, with a secondary purpose of showing a correlation between the individual's pain history and the situation of the lesions.

SIX CASE REPORTS

In our autopsy series there were 14 individuals with a history of whiplash injury and chronic pain. We have excluded from consideration three cases whose whiplash injury occurred more than 5 years before death (as it would have been too difficult to distinguish whiplash lesions from age changes), three cases who had undergone surgery for cervical interbody fusion and two cases where no whiplash lesions were found, leaving six cases with a theme of anterior annular disruption and rim lesions plus posterior disc herniations or protrusions.

   Most of the deaths in these 14 individuals were from drug overdoses of prescription narcotics associated with the individual's chronic pain and depression. In the two cases where no lesions were found, the predominant picture was one of long-term depression with associated chronic pain. One assumes that the three individuals who had surgical fusions would have had pain and pathology relating to the single segment that was fused, but after interbody fusions they continued to suffer from chronic pain.

   The six cases presented all have a history of whiplash injury between 1 and 5 years before death. Five were young adults unlikely to show age-related degenerative changes. The situation of the lesions correlated with, or was compatible with, the history of the patients' pain. Our case report findings support the view that most patients with chronic whiplash-associated disorder have lesions that account for their pain, adding credence to the view of Bogduk and others that many of these chronic pain patients have treatable lesions (Bogduk, 2006; Curatolo et al., 2011).

Case 1

A 30-year-old man sitting in a stationary sedan was hit from behind at about 60 km per hour. He suffered a neck extension whiplash injury with immediate onset of neck pain, occipital headache and recurrent 'shooting pains' down his right arm from the shoulder to the lateral forearm and whole hand. Examination found tenderness in the right trapezius and suprascapular region but no neurological signs. X-rays showed mild torticollis but no fractures; they also showed normal disc spaces.

   Treatment with non-steroidal anti-inflammatory drugs (NSAIDs) and physiotherapy did not alleviate the symptoms. Reviews at 4 months and 7 months noted persistent right shoulder pain, with pain and paraesthesia radiating down the right lateral arm to the whole hand including the ulnar digits. The patient also had occasional episodes of headache and blurred vision and his attempts to return to work were unsuccessful. X-rays at 7 months post-injury found newly developed ossicles in the anterior annulus at C4–5· and C5–6. Specialist review at 7 months described 'a mild cervical strain injury with muscle pain that would require a few more months to stabilise or resolve'. A physiotherapist reported 'clinical evidence of disc injuries'. GP review at 1 year reported persistence of moderate pain in the same distribution as before. The patient sought help from other sources but unexpectedly died 14 months after his injury.

   At autopsy his cervical spine was sectioned in 2.5 mm slices in the sagittal plane and sections were stained by the bone dye Alizarin. Rim lesions were found in the midline section of the discs and in parasagittal sections on the right side of the midline, present in all discs from C4–5 to C7–T1. No lesions were found in the facet joints. The rim lesions in all discs from C4–5 to C7–T1 were mainly on the right side and correlated very well with the patient's pain distribution from the C4 to the C8 dermatomes. Three of these lesions are illustrated in sagittal section in Figures 8.1 to 8.3.

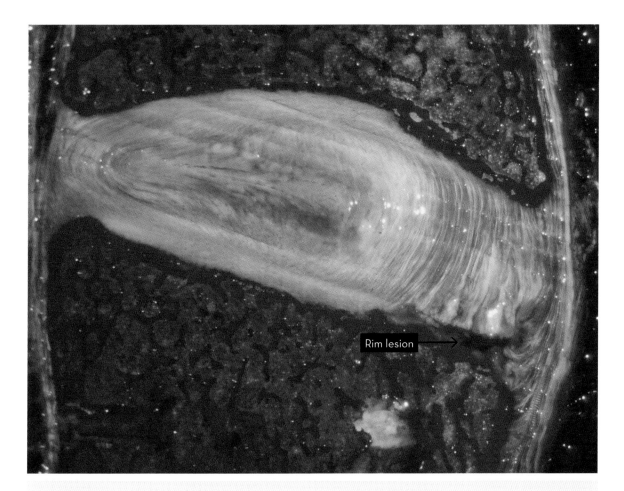

Rim lesion

FIGURE 8.1

Case 1: Rim lesion.

C4–5 shows a rim lesion in the lower anterior disc in a sagittal section stained by the bone dye Alizarin. (There is artefact light reflection from the surface of the section as it was not completely immersed in water. There is also a speck of saw-cut debris on the surface of C5.)

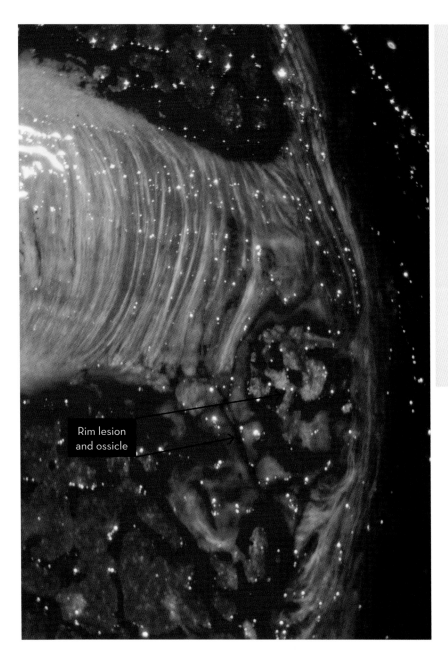

Rim lesion
and ossicle

FIGURE 8.2A
Case 1: Rim lesion and ossicle.

The sagittal section of the anterior part of C5–6; an ossicle has developed adjacent to a rim lesion in the anterior annulus. X-rays in the acute stage did not show any disc pathology but 7 months after the injury ossicles began to appear in the anterior annulus of both C4–5 and C5–6. The rim lesion lies between the ossicle and the vertebral body below.

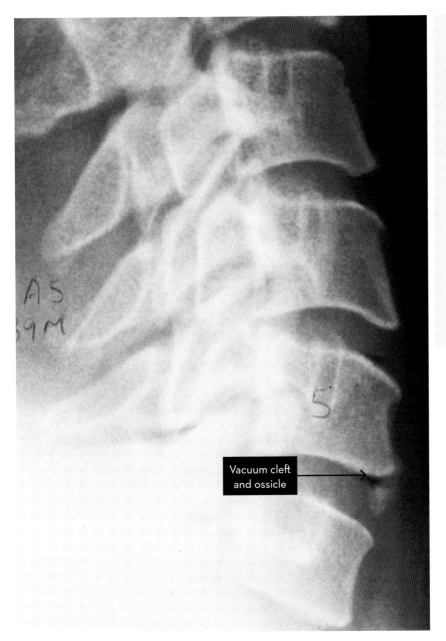

Vacuum cleft
and ossicle

FIGURE 8.2B
Case 1: Rim lesion and ossicle in a patient.

This lateral x-ray in extension is from a different, living patient with whiplash who had a similar response to injury of ossification adjacent to a rim lesion or vacuum cleft in the anterior annulus. Once again, the ossicle did not appear until some months after the whiplash injury.

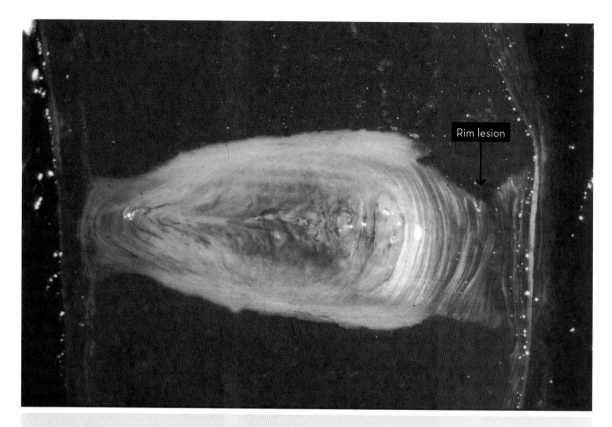

Rim lesion

FIGURE 8.3
Case 1: Rim lesion.

The C6–7 disc shows a rim lesion in the upper anterior disc. The disc is otherwise well-preserved.

Case 2

A 42-year-old woman suffered chronic pain for 3 years from injuries sustained in a left-side impact car accident at high speed. After the accident she had immediate onset of right-sided neck and head pain. By 1 month she had developed pain along the lateral aspect of her right upper limb with numbness and paraesthesia in her middle and ring fingers. She also had occipitotemporal headaches and complained of dizziness, blurred vision, an inability to concentrate and feeling faint. X-rays showed normal cervical spine alignment with slight narrowing of C4–5 and C5–6. A CT scan showed a minimal posterior bulge of C4–5.

A later MRI showed disc bulges at C3–4 and C4–5 and a marked protrusion at C5–6 with local flattening of the spinal cord. She showed painful restriction of all neck movements, anterior tenderness over C5–6 and 'global weakness' of her right arm with a strongly positive brachial plexus stretch test.

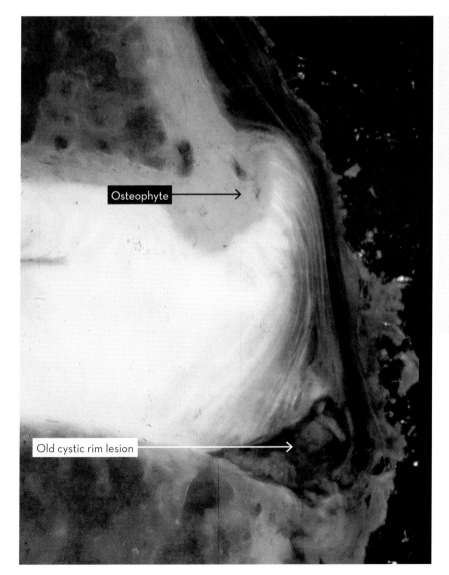

FIGURE 8.4

Case 2: A sagittal section of the anterior part of the C5–6 disc.

The large cystic rim lesion in the anterior annulus of C5–6 is a longstanding lesion probably from the car accident 3 years earlier. There is an osteophyte projecting down from the anterior margin of the C5 vertebral body into the injured anterior annulus of C5–6.

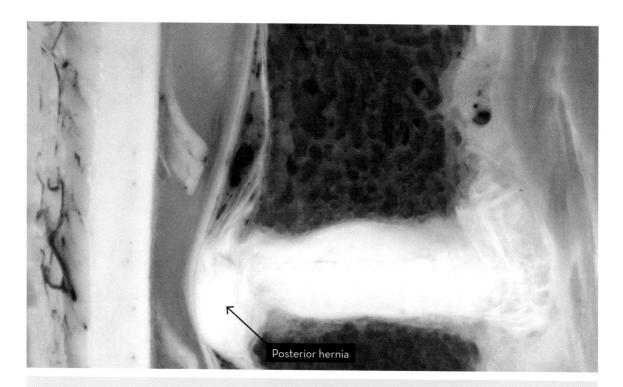

Posterior hernia

FIGURE 8.5
Case 2: Severe disc injury as shown in sagittal section.

A closer view of a right-sided parasagittal section shows the large posterolateral herniation at C5–6, which balloons the posterior longitudinal ligament backwards and narrows the spinal canal.

Case 3

A 26-year-old man had a motor cycle accident causing whiplash with neck pain referred to his right upper limb and occipital headaches. X-rays and a CT scan showed 'minimal traumatic damage' at C5–6 with partial facet subluxation. His severe neck pain, headaches and right arm pain persisted, requiring strong analgesics. Rehabilitation was unsuccessful. He became depressed and fatally overdosed with narcotics 3 years later. Sagittal sections at autopsy show the tissue responses to injury 3 years after this patient's neck trauma (Figure 8.6).

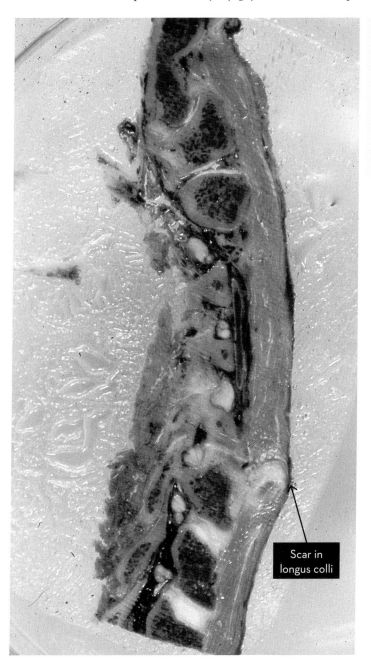

Scar in longus colli

FIGURE 8.6A

Case 3. A transverse scar in the longus colli muscle at the C5–6 level seen in sagittal section.

The scar indicates repair of a tear in the muscle at the time of the whiplash injury.

Figure 8.6 continues

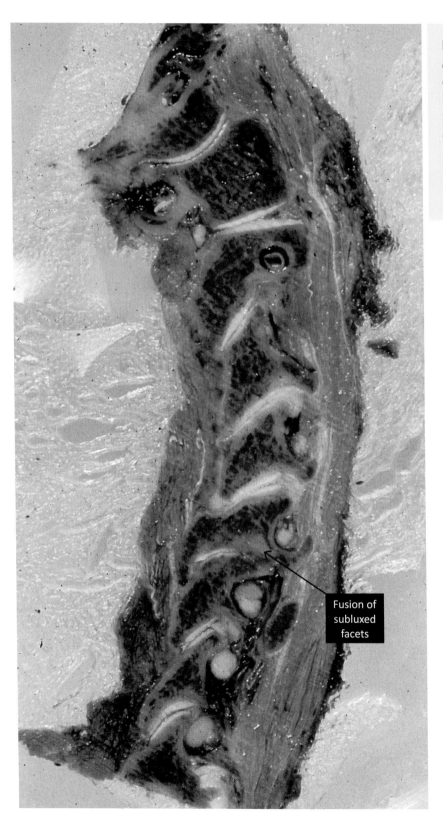

Fusion of
subluxed
facets

FIGURE 8.6B
Case 3. A subluxed C5 facet joint seen in parasagittal section.

This section shows a subluxed C5–6 facet joint with fusion across the anterior part of the joint.

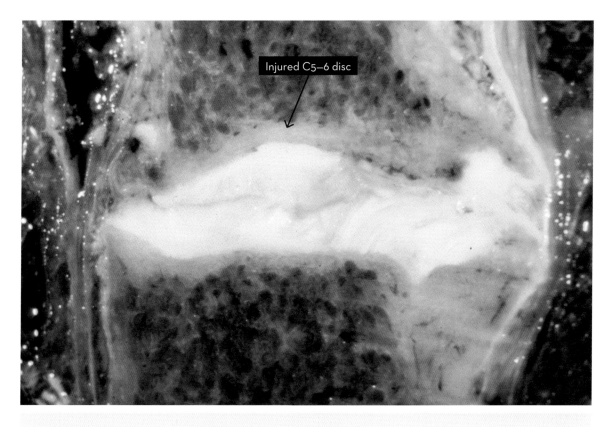

Injured C5–6 disc

FIGURE 8.6C
Case 3. Long-term disc changes following injury.

There is severe degeneration and distortion in the C5–6 disc with added new bone formation at the anterior surface. Judging by the changes in the disc and facet, the severity of this patient's original 'minor' injuries was underestimated. (Anterior is to the right.)

Case 4

A 58-year-old man suffered chronic pain from head and neck injuries sustained during a motor vehicle accident; he died 2 years later.

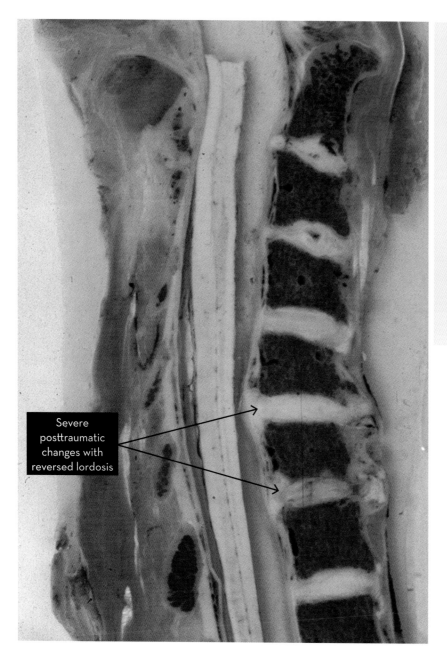

Severe posttraumatic changes with reversed lordosis

FIGURE 8.7

Case 4: A mid-sagittal section shows a posterior disc herniation at C5–6 with a sharply angled reversal of lordosis.

The C6–7 disc also shows severe posttraumatic degenerative changes and there are large anterior herniations of the C5–6 and C6–7 discs. The spinal cord is normal. (Anterior is to the right.)

Case 5

A 43-year-old man had a history of pain from a road accident causing whiplash. At the time of the injury he complained of neck pain, headache and paraesthesia in both arms and an inability to micturate; his bladder was enlarged to the umbilicus. He had decreased pin-prick sensation on the dorsolateral aspects of both upper limbs and marked neck tenderness, maximal at C4–5.

X-rays reported 'degenerative' loss of height in the C4–5 disc. The initial diagnosis was of 'whiplash' with minor nerve root symptoms, but his neck and arm pain persisted along with vertigo, altered consciousness, 'drop attacks' and weakness in both arms. Further x-rays were reported as normal. He had two brief hospital admissions when examination by a spinal surgeon suggested a minor central cord syndrome, and on lumbar puncture a neurosurgeon reported a cerebrospinal fluid (CSF) block when his neck was extended. However, other specialists suggested 'very strong functional elements in his symptoms'.

The patient's compensation case was settled 5 years later, but in court a surgeon for the insurance company and the judge were both critical of the patient's 'exaggeration of symptoms'. He was depressed and died of a drug overdose shortly after settlement.

At autopsy the Professor of Neuropathology found posterior interbody fusion at C4–5 (not reported on the patient's x-rays) and an old disc herniation on the left side. The posttraumatic interbody fusion did not affect his pain. The Professor also reported spinal cord distortion due to deformity of the canal at C4 with fibrous thickening of the meninges, as well as loss of myelinated fibres with dense gliosis of the left lateral column, consistent with a traumatic Brown-Sequard syndrome. The case was publicised by the late Sir George Bedbrook as a caution to colleagues not to overlook significant physical injuries due to an overemphasis on 'functional elements' in diagnosis.

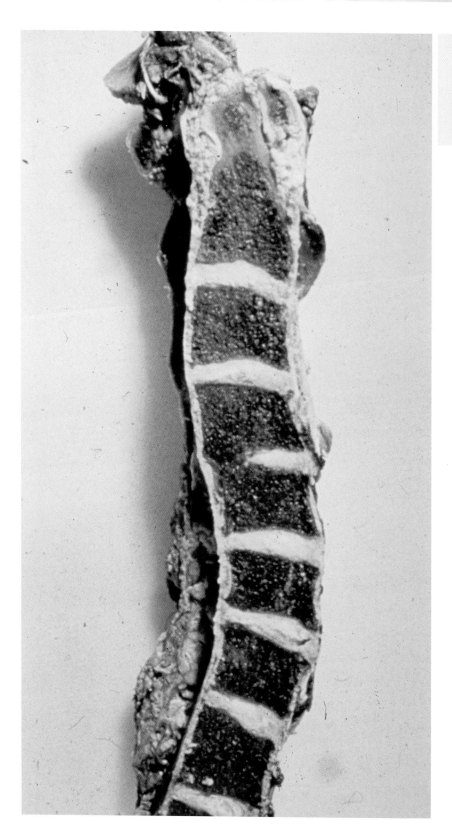

FIGURE 8.8
Case 5: A midline section showing late posttraumatic fusion at C4–5.

Case 6

A 24-year-old man was injured in a motor vehicle accident. He reported being violently shaken about by the 'forceful' impact from behind. He almost immediately developed neck pain with pain and paraesthesia in his left forearm and hand (C6, C7 and C8 dermatomes). He was treated without success and the severe occipitofrontal headaches and forearm/hand pain became chronic. His symptoms suggested a left carpal tunnel syndrome but nerve conduction tests were normal and there were 'few objective signs'. He was unable to resume work and lost his job. He died of an overdose of prescription narcotics aged 27.

At autopsy, rim lesions and cystic changes were found in both the C6–7 and C7–T1 anterior annulus. There was also articular cartilage loss in both C6–7 and C7–T1 facet joints with marginal osteophytes.

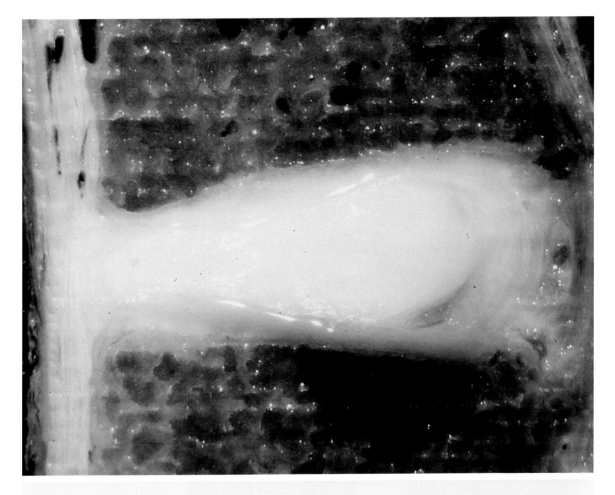

FIGURE 8.9A

Case 6: Cystic changes in the anterior annulus as seen in sagittal section.

Cystic disruption of the anterior annulus of the C6–7 disc. There were similar less severe changes in the C7–T1 disc.

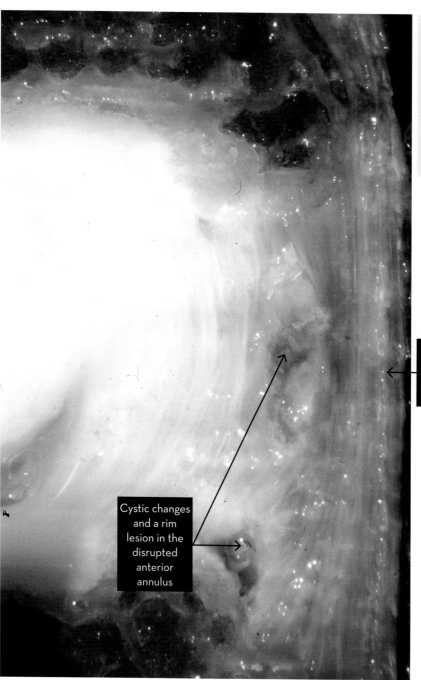

FIGURE 8.9B
Case 6: Posttraumatic changes in the anterior annulus including a cystic rim lesion and other cystic changes.

The anterior longitudinal ligament is intact

Cystic changes and a rim lesion in the disrupted anterior annulus

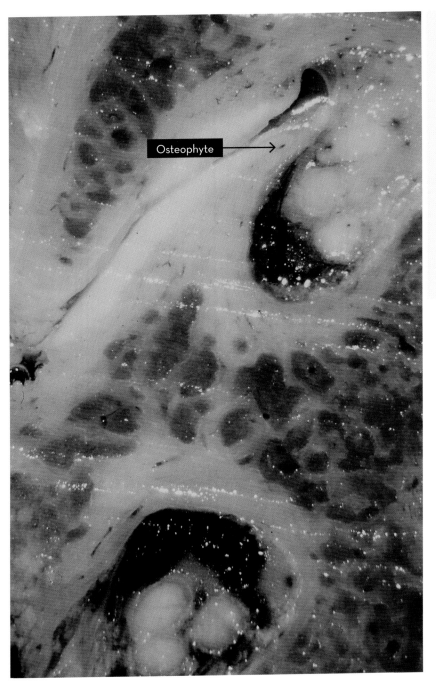

Osteophyte

FIGURE 8.10

Case 6: Arthritic changes in a facet joint, shown in sagittal section.

Arthritic changes in the left C7–T1 facet joint, including partial loss of the articular cartilage and the growth of a large anterior osteophyte impinging on the C8 nerve roots. (Anterior is to the right.)

ADDITIONAL CASE

In our autopsy study of 14 subjects with a history of chronic whiplash pain, three were rejected from analysis because they had undergone surgical interbody fusion. The fusion would have been performed at the most painful, injured level. Unfortunately, the three surgical fusions appeared to be unsuccessful in giving significant pain relief. An interbody fusion with a graft is shown in Figure 8.11. Jonsson and colleagues (1994) claimed that in 10 patients with large disc herniations on MRI, discectomy and fusion gave pain relief.

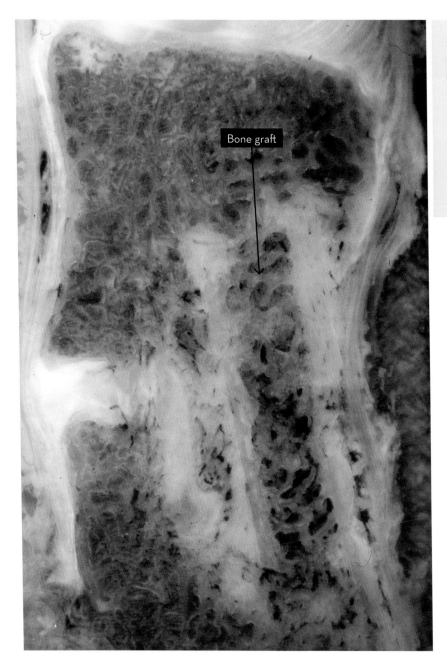

FIGURE 8.11

Surgical interbody fusion, with a successful bone graft as seen in sagittal section.

Unfortunately, the patient continued to suffer neck pain and headache.

Bone graft

VASCULAR CONGESTION IN SUBOCCIPITAL VEINS AS A POSSIBLE CAUSE OF POST-WHIPLASH HEADACHES

A finding of interest and possible significance in these post-whiplash cases is the frequency of venous engorgement in the suboccipital space. Sagittal sections of Cases 3 and 6 show marked vascular proliferation and engorgement behind the C1–2 lateral joint, around the C2 nerve roots. These changes may relate to occipital headaches. The images in Figure 8.12 are of Case 6. Similar vascular congestion was also found in the suboccipital region in the autopsies of two other chronic whiplash individuals.

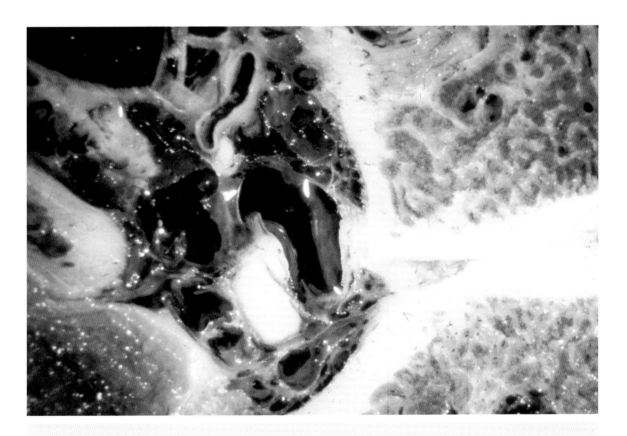

FIGURE 8.12A

Case 6: Vascular proliferation and engorgement behind the C1–2 lateral joint, around the C2 nerve roots.

The dorsal root ganglion is surrounded by large, dilated veins.

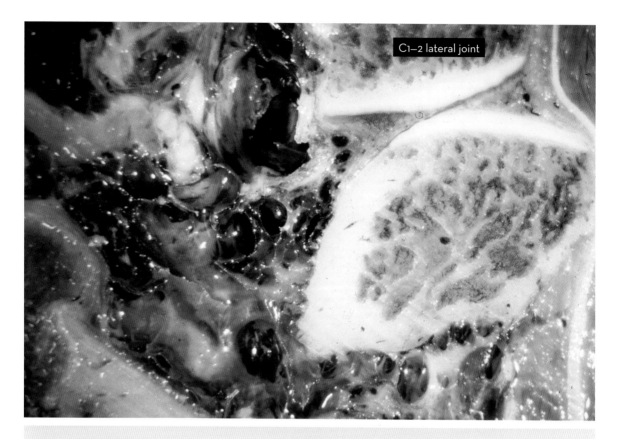

C1–2 lateral joint

FIGURE 8.12B

Case 6: Another example of vascular proliferation and engorgement behind the C1–2 lateral joint, around the C2 nerve roots.

The suboccipital venous plexus is at a confluence of valveless veins including vertebral veins, epidural veins from the anterior spinal canal and deep cervical veins. Congestion in the suboccipital veins has been implicated as a possible cause of occipital headaches (Jansen et al., 1989).

THE SUBOCCIPITAL VENOUS PLEXUS AND VASCULAR HEADACHES

Chronic headaches in whiplash-associated disorder have been attributed to varicosity in the suboccipital venous plexus with irritation of the C2 nerve. Jansen and colleagues (1989) claimed to have cured chronic occipital headaches in 16 patients by removing these veins. Pikus and Phillips (1995) used similar 'decompression' of the C2 nerve roots in the treatment of cervicogenic headaches. We found an enlarged plexus of these veins at autopsy in patients who had a history of chronic occipital headaches. These valveless veins have widespread connections and blood can flow in varying directions. The largest contributors to the venous plexus are the paired longitudinal anterior epidural venous sinuses, which drain spinal structures: they join with vertebral veins and deep cervical veins in an anastomotic network of thin-walled veins behind C1 and C2 where they are partly enclosed in a compartment below the occipital bone and deep to the inferior oblique muscle. When they are congested they fill this compartmental suboccipital space. The suboccipital venous plexus was described by Wesley Parke (1978) as being unique, in that small arterioles fed into the veins creating a higher venous pressure than normal around the second cervical dorsal root ganglion and the origin of the greater occipital nerve.

ARE BLUNT TRAUMA INJURIES FROM FATAL CAR ACCIDENTS COMPARABLE WITH WHIPLASH INJURIES IN SURVIVORS OF CAR ACCIDENTS?

It is argued that the blunt trauma of a fatal car accident is generally much greater than that causing whiplash injury in survivors, but various studies suggest that there is considerable overlap. Patients who survive with quadriplegia have more severe spinal injuries than those shown in this atlas, where we have deliberately focused on lesions in well-aligned spines rather than gross fracture dislocations in order to study possible whiplash injuries. Studies of injuries in cadaver spines and experimental injuries in animals show that the injuries can occur with levels of violence comparable to fatal car accidents (Taylor & Twomey, 2005).

Frontal impacts greater than 8 G produce ligamentous injuries in cadaver necks (Panjabi et al., 1998) and Macnab's (1973) classical experimental studies of rear-end impact neck injuries in primates designed the forces to mimic whiplash and showed that this produced similar injuries to those illustrated in this atlas. Other recent studies of forces involved in frontal collisions confirm disc failure at 22 G (Panzer, Fice & Cronin, 2011). It follows that much lower G forces would be likely to injure cervical structures in a rear-end or side-impact collision (Pearson, Ivancic & Panjabi, 2004; Erbulut, 2014). Murray Alan (1997), from his tests in volunteers, suggests likely thresholds for pain of 8, 16 and 24 km per hour for rear, side and frontal impacts, respectively (see also Taylor & Twomey, 2005).

ARE NECK INJURIES SECONDARY TO HEAD IMPACT COMPARABLE WITH THOSE WITHOUT EVIDENCE OF HEAD IMPACT?

Neck injuries resulting from head impacts were predominantly the case in our study. But we compared these injuries with the injuries of those who died of torso injuries with no external evidence of head impact. There was a greater frequency of dens fractures, atlanto-occipital dislocations and C1–2 soft-tissue injuries in subjects with severe head injuries than in those with fatal torso injuries. However, the subaxial injuries (C2 to T1) were similar in nature and segmental distribution comparing the head injuries with the torso injuries.

WHIPLASH LESIONS IN PATIENTS COMPARED WITH AUTOPSY LESIONS: VACUUM CLEFTS AND RIM LESIONS

Despite the difficulty of demonstrating soft-tissue lesions in whiplash patients, due to the reliance on plain x-rays, vacuum clefts are not uncommon in whiplash patients when lateral x-rays are done in extension. Vacuum clefts were found in whiplash patients in our pain clinic, but they only showed up in lateral x-rays with the neck in extension. A brief search of clinic records for patients with whiplash injuries who had had lateral x-rays in extension uncovered 15 patients with clefts in the anterior annulus. One example was found on CT scan (Figure 8.13A). The clefts were in exactly the same situation as the acute rim lesions in our blunt trauma study and were similar in situation to the chronic rim lesions in Case 1. The age range of the 15 patients was 19–49 years, with an average age of 35. Vacuum clefts have traditionally been regarded as degenerative changes when found in middle-aged or elderly patients with no whiplash history, but their strong association with acute whiplash lesions in young adults suggests that the clefts found in these 15 patients are whiplash lesions. References in the literature to 'lucent clefts' relate them to whiplash injuries (see Bohrer & Chea, 1988; Miller et al., 1978; Reymond et al., 1972; Cheong & Tan, 1991; Waxman & Rizzo, 1996).

In our blunt trauma study rim lesions were seen most often at segments where high facet angles exposed discs to high shearing forces. Lumbar rim lesions were cited by Osti, Vernon-Roberts and Fraser (1990) as precursors of degenerative changes in lumbar discs.

Examples of cervical vacuum clefts are shown in Figure 8.13A and B. The CT scan shows the lateral spread of the cleft on each side of the midline. The rim lesions shown in sagittal section in Case 1 (Figures 8.1–8.3) also spread to the right and left of the midline.

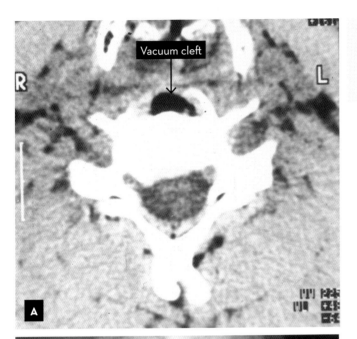

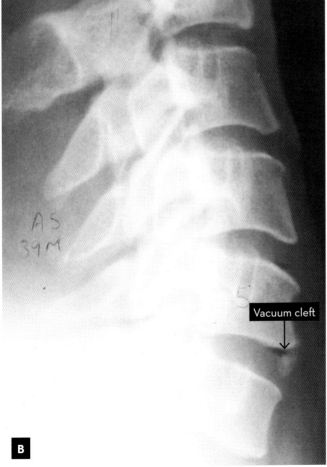

FIGURE 8.13A and B
Vacuum clefts.

(A) CT scan. **(B)** X-ray extension view.

SEVERE DISC INJURIES

Posterior disc herniations are often found in patients with severe whiplash injuries. They were commonly found in our blunt trauma study and also in our case report study. The only lesions commonly found in our acute blunt trauma study but rarely seen in chronic whiplash patients were linear disc avulsions from the vertebral body in young adults and severe disc disruptions in older patients. Avulsion injuries may be identified only in acute trauma, while in chronic whiplash-associated injury such injuries may change into severe degenerative disc changes including vertebral body fusions across the injured discs, as seen in Cases 2, 3 and 5. Uhrenholt, Grunnet-Nilsson and Hartvigsen (2002) drew attention to the observation that whiplash patients whose discs appear normal or only slightly reduced in the acute stage develop more severe changes in the succeeding years.

Various authors have investigated disc injuries resulting from trauma including whiplash:

- Jomin and colleagues (1986) surveyed a large series of disc herniations, most of them from trauma
- Pettersson, Hildingsson and Toolanen (1997), using magnetic resonance tomography, found posterior herniations in 13 of 39 of their young adult acute whiplash patients
- Davis and colleagues (1991) demonstrated rim lesions and disc herniations in whiplash cases on MRI
- Anderson and colleagues (2012) identified MRI findings significantly associated with whiplash injuries
- Otremski and colleagues (1989) and Sivola and colleagues (2002) also identified disc injuries in whiplash patients.

We found posterior disc herniations in a small proportion of chronic whiplash patents but they were the most common severe disc injuries in living patients.

Examples of these disc injuries are shown in Figures 8.14A, B and C.

EXAMPLES OF DISC LESIONS IN PATIENTS

Example 1

A young woman who suffered a whiplash injury in a car accident presented 4 years later with chronic neck pain, disability and a history of depression. At the time of her injury, a C6 radiculopathy had been diagnosed, but plain x-rays were reported normal and no further investigations were pursued. Her pain became chronic and she became severely depressed.

At her 4-year review, she had symptoms and signs suggestive of a C5–6 pain source with local pain and tenderness at C5–6 both anteriorly and posteriorly. Examination of a series of her neck x-rays taken at intervals since the injury found a subtle but consistent flattening of an uncinate process at C6 in all films (Figure 8.14A). An MRI was ordered, which found a C5–6 disc herniation impinging on and flattening the cord with a posterior annular tear (Figure 8.14B and C). Her eventual diagnosis of a physical injury at C5–6 made it easier for her to come to terms with her pain and removed her sense of guilt and self-blame that it was 'all in her head'. Her symptoms improved considerably with reassurance and conservative management and she later responded well to C5–6 facet neurotomy.

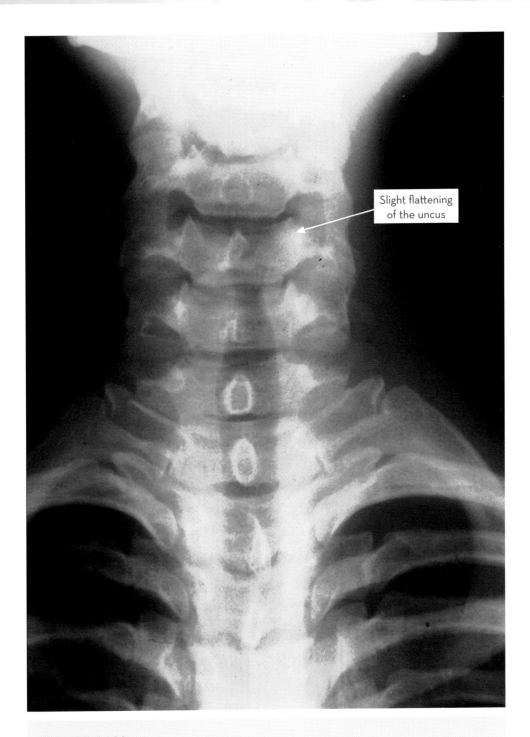

Slight flattening of the uncus

FIGURE 8.14A

Example 1. Flattening and asymmetry of an uncinate process at C6.

The patient had pain and tenderness at C5–6 and proved to have a disc herniation (Figure 8.14B and C).

Figure 8.14 continues

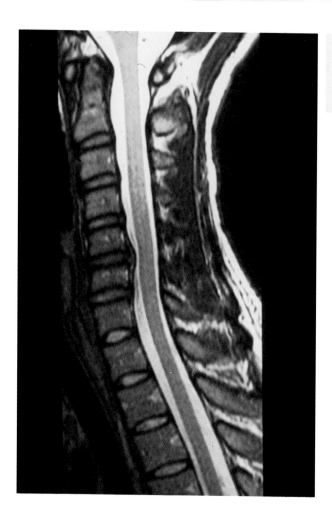

FIGURE 8.14B

Example 1. A C5–6 disc herniation with concordant symptoms.

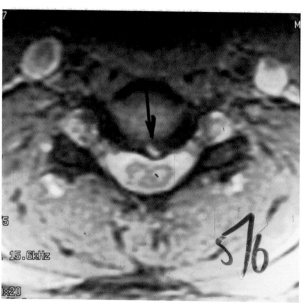

FIGURE 8.14C

Example 1. A posterior annular tear.

The C5–6 disc herniation has flattened the spinal cord. The high signal area is reported as a posterior annular tear (see arrow).

Example 2

A 26-year-old woman with chronic whiplash-associated disorder suffered from chronic neck pain and headaches after a motor vehicle accident. The severity of her symptoms merited an MRI scan (Figure 8.15). Conservative management had only limited success in relieving her pain.

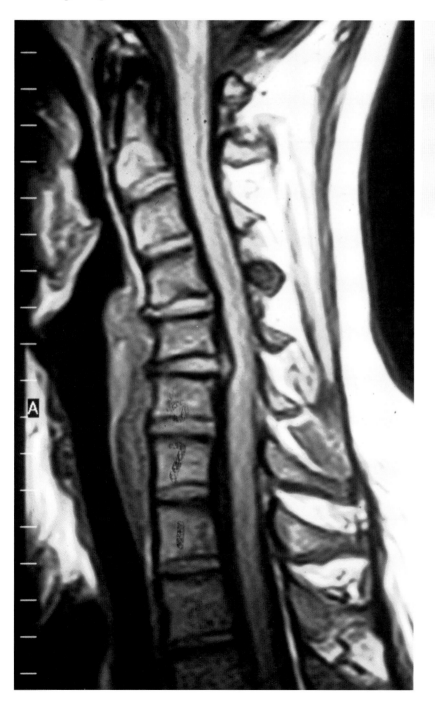

FIGURE 8.15

Example 2: A C5–6 herniation indenting the cord with reversal of lordosis.

A high signal region in the bulging anterior annulus at C4–5 was suggestive of a rim lesion.

FACET PAIN AND LESIONS

Persistent nociception in a cervical facet joint has been convincingly demonstrated in many studies, citing concordant responses to injections using both long- and short-acting anaesthetic blocks and placebo (Lord et al., 1996; MacVicar et al., 2012; Engel et al., 2016) but without demonstration of the responsible lesions.

Our blunt trauma study illustrates a wide variety of both soft-tissue lesions and fractures (undisplaced) that were easily identified on sectioning at autopsy but that were usually missed on postmortem x-rays. Likewise, standard x-rays of living patients with local pain, marked focal tenderness and dysfunction in a specific facet joint rarely show an injury to the joint on x-ray examination. Yet these same patients often show 'hot spots' on bone scan with SPECT (single-photon emission computed tomography) corresponding with the clinical findings in the symptomatic joint.

ZYGAPOPHYSEAL FACET 'HOT SPOTS'

When zygapophyseal facet 'hot spots' are demonstrated by bone scans they suggest 'healing' whiplash injuries. It has been widely claimed that chronic whiplash pain originates most often (54%) in the facet joints (Barnsley, Lord & Bogduk, 1994). Soft-tissue injuries are not demonstrated by x-rays and undisplaced fractures are readily missed as lateral views superimpose both articular columns. Technetium bone scans can demonstrate 'healing activity' in injured facets, and in young people without degenerative changes a bone scan with tomography can demonstrate an injury in a symptomatic joint.

Clinical correlation with bone scans

We surveyed 22 young adult patients to test the clinical correlation with bone scans (Figures 8.16 and 8.17). An expert manipulative physiotherapist (Robert Elvey) and the author undertook blind examinations, locating painful, dysfunctional facet joints in whiplash patients with chronic pain: 37 of 49 clinically painful and dysfunctional facet joints showed increased bone scan activity; however, 9 asymptomatic joints also showed some increased activity (Cardaci, Bower & Taylor, 1999).

Bone scans can provide useful confirmation of a healing injury in a painful joint, but bone scan changes in older subjects may not be attributable to injury. The bone scan findings must be taken together with other evidence in reaching a diagnosis.

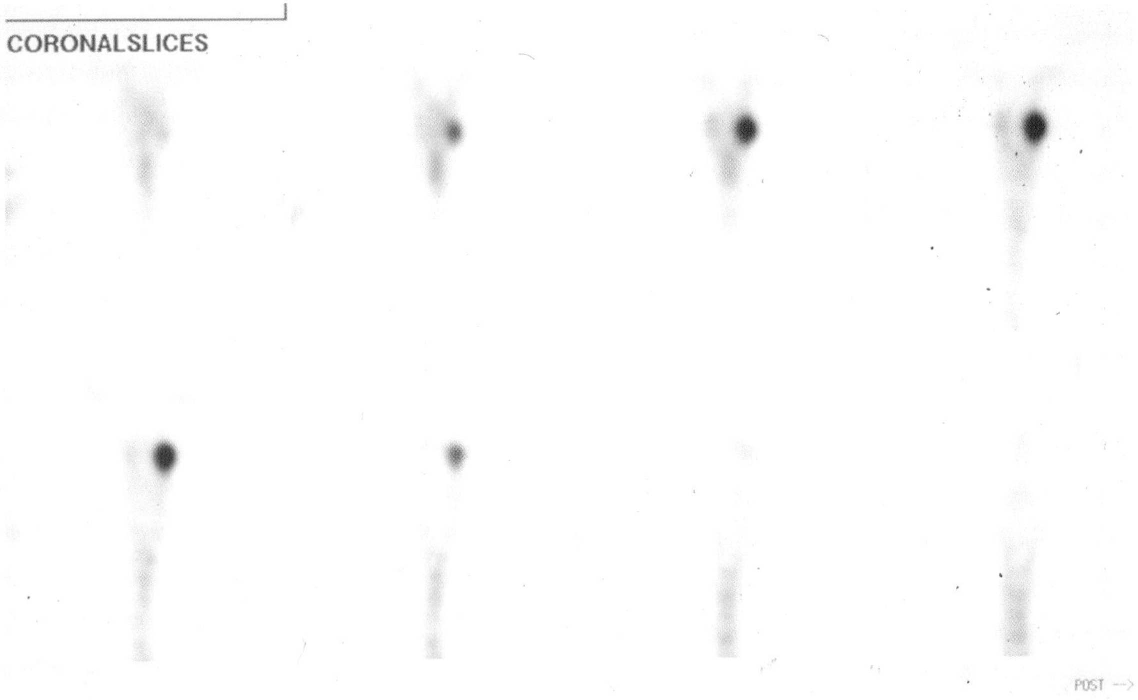

CORONAL SLICES

POST —>

FIGURE 8.16

A young man with pain, tenderness and dysfunction at C2–3 on clinical examination showed a 'hot spot' in the same joint on the bone scan.

The coronal sections from the single-photon emission computed tomography (SPECT) demonstrate a 'hot spot' at the same joint.

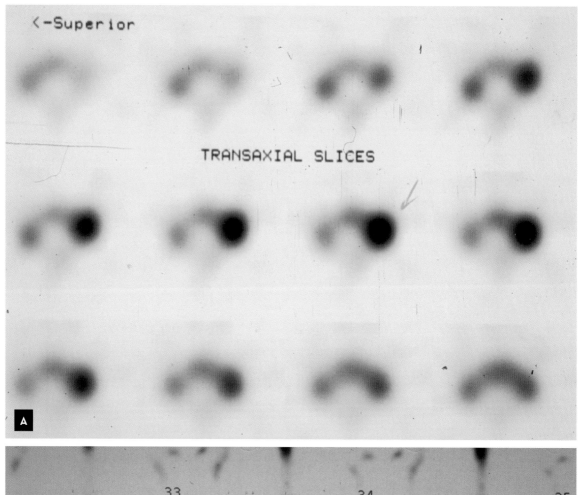

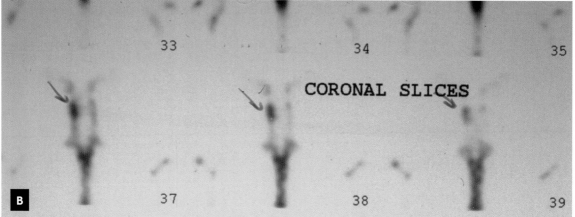

FIGURE 8.17A and B

Bone scans from two young patients show good correlation between clinical findings and the sites of 'hot spots' in the scans.

(A) Transaxial slices show strong activity suggestive of a healing fracture (see arrow).
(B) Coronal slices show a clearly demonstrated 'hot spot' (see arrows).

SUMMARY AND CONCLUSIONS

This atlas of anatomy, age changes and injuries is based on careful examination and photography of serial sections of 266 cervical spines, covering the whole age range from early childhood to old age. We are unaware of any comparable study apart from the excellent, but smaller, study of 22 injured spines by Jonsson and colleagues (1991).

Upper cervical joints

Sagittal sectioning of the upper cervical synovial joints demonstrates with clarity the fine structural features of their articular cartilages and synovium. The Co–1 lateral joints are congruous, while the C1–2 lateral joints are biconvex with large synovial folds filling the anterior and posterior marginal spaces. These triangular vascular synovial folds are vulnerable to injury in sudden forceful movements such as in a car accident. The dens is the fulcrum for a large part of cervical axial rotation and it is noted that the upper cervical movements of flexion, extension and axial rotation are often well preserved in old age when degenerative changes in the subaxial joints make them stiff. The progressive stiffness of the subaxial cervical spine with ageing makes the upper levels more vulnerable to life-threatening injury in falls or other blunt trauma.

Normal subaxial anatomy and age changes

This atlas demonstrates unique features of the cervical spine, the most slender and mobile part of the vertebral column with its particular vulnerability to trauma, especially trauma in extension. The cervical spine pays a price for its wide range of motion in the progressive, early adult fissuring of its intervertebral discs. Uncovertebral clefts appear in later childhood or early adolescence in the narrowest lateral intervertebral spaces, and in early adult life fissures spread medially from these clefts into the centres of the discs. In middle-aged and elderly individuals we often noted the development of postero-lateral uncovertebral and posterior marginal osteophytes. The osteophytes crowd or entrap the nerve roots at their exit from the spinal canal through the intervertebral foramina. The large dorsal root ganglia of the brachial plexus (C5–T1) are especially affected. We show how the peripheral bulging of discs and osteophytes deforms the originally straight vertebral arteries to make them tortuous and how cervical spinal stenosis may be caused by the posterior protrusion of discs and marginal osteophytes into the spinal canal.

Disc injuries

The portrayal of the normal structure of discs at different ages forms the basis for recognition of traumatic changes, especially along the relatively weak linear junction of the vertebral bodies with the disc. Our study demonstrates the high frequency of acute tears of the anterior annulus away from the vertebral rim (rim lesions). These acute tears, resulting from blunt trauma, show spread of blood from the tear between the annular lamellae. The anterior longitudinal ligament remains intact. The traumatic clefts persist and may become cystic in later years in patients with a history of whiplash who later die from other causes. They correspond to the vacuum clefts described in living patients with a history of whiplash (Bohrer & Chea, 1988; Miller et al., 1978; Cheong & Tan, 1991).

In more severe trauma we found linear avulsions of discs away from their normal attachment to the vertebral bodies and posterior disc herniations that usually leave the posterior longitudinal ligament intact, tenting it backwards. MRI studies seeking to clarify the nature of whiplash injuries have not found the range of disc injuries shown in this atlas, although they agree with our findings of disc herniation (Davis et al., 1991; Pettersson et al., 1997; Sivola et al., 2002; Vetti et al., 2011; Anderson et al., 2012).

Zygapophyseal facet joints

Facet joint anatomy and pathology are well shown in sagittal section. The paucity or absence of a posterior fibrous capsule allows intimate contact of the posterior joint synovium with the covering deep fibres of the multifidus. This absence of a fibrous capsule is a feature characteristic of highly mobile joints. Facet joints do not degenerate as early as the corresponding discs, but loss of disc height with ageing adversely affects facet biomechanics and they may become arthritic. Their articular cartilages lose thickness with age and they develop marginal osteophytes.

The normal and age change studies lay the foundation for recognition and description of soft-tissue injuries to facet joints in blunt whiplash-type trauma, injuries that are missed with current imaging techniques in living subjects. These soft-tissue injuries in cervical facet joints, as well as minor undisplaced facet fractures, have been suspected for many years (Bogduk, 2006; Curatolo et al., 2011; Lord et al., 1996; Uhrenholt, Grunnet-Nilsson & Hartvigsen, 2002) but rarely demonstrated. Despite demonstrating a wide range of facet injuries to capsular structures and articular cartilages in our autopsy studies, and despite our clinical findings of focal facet tenderness and dysfunction, our imaging investigations in whiplash patients failed to show many facet injuries, but in the same patients bone scans with SPECT frequently demonstrated obvious 'hot spots' due to healing activity in the painful tender facet joints. We have reviewed the studies that show that it is possible to observe the same lesions in experimental animals and in living patients as those observed at autopsy (see Taylor & Twomey, 2005).

Dorsal root ganglion injuries

One of the surprising findings in our study was the frequency of injury to dorsal root ganglia in up to a third of blunt trauma deaths. The injury was recognised most easily in those who survived long enough for continuing circulation to cause central bleeding in the acutely injured ganglia. This appeared to be a stretch injury, most obvious in side-impact motor vehicle accidents or in falls onto the head and shoulders, but also in extension injuries and in 'shaken babies'. A substantial proportion of injured ganglia with primary injuries to small blood vessels also showed axonal disruption. It is interesting to speculate whether the majority of whiplash patients with neuropathic pain may have suffered a dorsal root ganglion injury. Neuropathic pain is common in chronic whiplash-associated disorder and it seems likely that dorsal root ganglion injury may be a major contributor. The brachial plexus stretch test is regarded as a reliable test of nerve root irritation or injury and it is positive in many whiplash patients (Quintner, 1989; Hall & Elvey, 1999; Ide, Ide & Yamaga, 2001; Wainner et al., 2003).

Chronic pain and post-injury reactive changes

Our blunt trauma study demonstrates injuries likely to occur in whiplash and our case reports show chronic whiplash injuries. The pain of chronic whiplash-associated disorder is a complex issue. The development of both central and peripheral neural hypersensitivity and the frequent development of depressive illness complicate the relationship of the pain to the original injury. However, it is suggested, based on a number of studies, that the nervous system hypersensitivity and behavioural abnormalities of chronic whiplash-associated disorder are secondary to the persisting nociceptive pain from injured joints or other structures and that these reactive features are often reversible with effective pain relief (Engel et al., 2016; Schneider et al., 2010; Smith et al., 2014, 2016; Wallis et al., 1996).

Muscle atrophy

Changes in the deep muscles closely applied around injured joints, with atrophy and disordered movement, are another common accompaniment of chronic whiplash pain (Elliott et al., 2006; Elliott et al., 2014; Falla et al., 2004; Jull, 2000). Muscle atrophy in patients with chronic pain is not unique to the cervical spine. In 41 of 193 (21%) CT scans from patients with chronic low back pain we found signs of segmental instability associated in most cases with atrophy of the multifidus and replacement of muscle tissue by fat (Taylor & O'Sullivan, 2000). One would hope that these changes might be prevented, reduced or reversed by appropriate rehabilitation programs. Long-term changes in the deep muscles controlling the painful joint will require ongoing rehabilitation to reestablish normal muscle control of the painful joints (Jull et al., 2008a, 2008b).

BIBLIOGRAPHY

Abram, SE, Yi, J, Fuchs, A & Hogan, QH 2006 Permeability of injured and intact peripheral nerves and dorsal root ganglia. *Anasthesiology*, 105, pp. 146–153.

Allen, M 1997 *Physical Medicine Research Foundation's BC Whiplash Initiative*. Instructor Handbook, Physical Medicine Research Foundation, Canada, pp. 1–95.

Anderson, S, Boesch, C, Zimmerman, H et al. 2012 Are there cervical spine findings at MR imaging that are specific to acute symptomatic whiplash injury? A prospective controlled study. *Radiology*, 262, pp. 567–575.

Aprill, C & Bogduk, N 1990 The accuracy of pain maps in predicting a pain source. *Spine*, 15, p. 458.

Barnsley, L, Lord, S & Bogduk, N 1994 Whiplash injury. *Pain*, 58, pp. 283–307.

Bogduk, N 2006 Editorial: Whiplash can have lesions. *Pain Research and Management*, 11, p. 155.

Bogduk, N & Aprill, C 1993 On the nature of neck pain, discography and cervical zygapophysial joint blocks. *Pain*, 54, pp. 213–217.

Bohrer, S & Chea, Y 1988 Cervical spine annulus vacuum. *Skeletal Radiology*, 17, pp. 324–329.

Boyd-Clark, L, Briggs, C & Galea, M 2004 Segmental degeneration in the cervical spine and associated changes in the dorsal root ganglia. *Clinical Anatomy*, 17, pp. 468–477.

Cardaci, G, Bower, G & Taylor, J 1999 Optimized cervical spine bone SPECT for detection of facet joint injury after whiplash injury. *Nuclear Medicine Communications*, 20, p. 366.

Cheong, WY & Tan, KP 1991 Air in the cervical annulus: The lucent cleft sign. *Singapore Medical Journal*, 32, pp. 255–257.

Cloward, RB 1959 Cervical diskography. A contribution to the etiology and mechanism of neck, shoulder and arm pain. *Annals of Surgery*, 150, pp. 1052–1064.

Curatolo, C, Bogduk, N, Ivancic P et al. 2011 The role of tissue damage in whiplash-associated disorders. *Spine*, 255, pp. S309–S315.

Curatolo, M, Arendt-Nilsen, L & Peterson-Felis, S 2004 Evidence, mechanisms and clinical implications of central hypersensitivity in chronic pain after whiplash injury. *Clinical Journal of Pain*, 20, pp. 469–476.

Davis, S, Teresi, L, Bradley, WG et al. 1991 Cervical spine hyperextension injuries: MR findings. *Radiology*, 180, pp. 245–251.

Dwyer, AC, Bogduk, N & Aprill, C 1990 Cervical zygapophyseal joint pain patterns. I. A study in normal volunteers. *Spine*, 15, p. 453.

Elliott, J 2011 The evidence for pathoanatomical lesions. In Sterling, M (ed.), *Whiplash: Evidence base for clinical practice*. Elsevier, Sydney.

Elliot, J, Jull, G, Noteboom, J et al. 2006 Fatty infiltration in cervical extensor muscles in persistent WAD. An MRI analysis. *Spine*, 31, pp. E846–E855.

Elliott, J, Pedler, AR, Jull, GA et al. 2014 Differential changes in muscle composition exist in traumatic and non-traumatic neck pain. *Spine*, 39, pp. 39–47.

Elvey, R 1986 Treatment of arm pain associated with abnormal brachial plexus tension. *Australian Journal of Physiotherapy*, 32, pp. 225–233.

Elvey, R 1997 Physical evaluation of the peripheral nervous system in disorders of pain and dysfunction. *Journal of Hand Therapy*, 10, pp. 122–129.

Engel, A, Rappard, G, King W et al. 2016 The effectiveness and risks of fluoroscopically guided cervical medial branch thermal radiofrequency neurotomy: A systemic review. *Pain Medicine*, 17, pp. 638–669.

Erbulut, DU 2014 Biomechanics of neck injuries resulting from rear-end vehicle collisions. *Turkish Neurosurgery*, 24, pp. 466–470.

Ettlin, TM, Kischka, U, Reichmann, S et al. 1992 Cerebral symptoms after whiplash injury of the neck: A prospective clinical and neuropsychological study of whiplash injury. *Journal of Neurology, Neurosurgery & Psychiatry*, 55, pp. 943–948.

Evans, RS 1992 Some observations on whiplash injuries. *Neurologic Clinics*, 10, pp. 975–997.

Falla, D, Jull, G & Hodges, P 2004 Patients with neck pain demonstrate reduced electromyographic activity of the deep cervical flexor muscles during performance of the craniocervical flexion test. *Spine*, 29, pp. 2108–2114.

Filler, A, Kliot, M, Howe, F et al. 1993 Application of magnetic resonance neurography in the evaluation of patients with peripheral nerve pathology. *The Lancet*, 341, pp. 659–661.

Finch, P & Taylor, J 1996 Functional anatomy of the spine. In Waldeman, S & Winnie, A (eds), *Interventional pain management*. Saunders, Philadelphia.

Fukui, S, Ohseto, K, Shiotani, M et al. 1996 Referred pain distribution of the cervical zygapophyseal joints and cervical dorsal rami. *Pain*, 68, pp. 79–83.

Giles, L & Taylor, J 1983 Histological preparation of large vertebral specimens. *Stain Technology*, 58, pp. 45–49.

Guez, M, Hildingsson, C, Rosengren, L et al. 2003 Neural markers in cerebrospinal fluid after cervical spine injuries and whiplash trauma. *Journal of Neurotrauma*, 20, pp. 853–858.

Hall, T & Elvey, R 1999 Nerve trunk pain: Physical diagnosis and treatment. *Manual Therapy*, 4, pp. 63–73.

Hallgren, R, Greenman, P & Rechtien, J 1994 Atrophy of sub-occiptial muscles in patients with chronic pain: A pilot study. *Journal of the American Osteopathic Association*, 94, pp. 1032–1038.

Head, J 1995 Morphology of the cervical spine and age-related changes. Honours BSc thesis, Curtin University, Perth.

Hirsch, C, Schazowitz, F & Galante, J 1967 Structural changes in the cervical spine. *Acta Orthopaedica Scandinavica*, Suppl 109, pp. 1–77.

Hoppenfeld, S 1976 *Physical examination of the spine and extremities.* Appleton Century Crofts/Prentice-Hall, New York.

Ibrahim, JE, Bugeja, L, Willoughby, M et al 2017 Premature deaths of nursing home residents: An epidemiological analysis. *Medical Journal of Australia*, 206(10), pp. 442–447.

Ide, M, Ide, J & Yamaga, M 2001 Symptoms and signs of irritation of the brachial plexus in whiplash injuries. *Journal of Bone & Joint Surgery*, 83B, pp. 226–229.

Jain, NB 2015 Traumatic spinal cord injury in USA, 1993–2012. *JAMA*, 313, pp. 2236–2243.

Jansen, J, Bardosi, A, Hildebrandt, J et al. 1989 Cervicogenic hemicranial attacks associated with vascular irritation of the cervical nerve root C2. *Pain*, 39, pp. 203–212.

Jomin, M, Lesoin, F, Lozes, G et al. 1986 Herniated cervical discs: Analysis of a series of 230 cases. Acta *Neurochirurgica*, 79, pp. 107–113.

Jonsson, H, Bring, G, Rauschning, W et al. 1991 Hidden cervical spine injuries in traffic accident victims with skull fractures. *Journal of Spinal Disorders*, 4, pp. 251–263.

Jonsson, H, Cesarini, K, Sahlstedt, B & Rauschning, W 1994 Findings and outcome in whiplash-type neck distortions. *Spine*, 19(24), pp. 2733–2743.

Jull, G 2000 Deep cervical flexor muscle dysfunction in whiplash. *Journal of Musculoskeletal Pain*, 8, pp. 143–145.

Jull, G, Bogduk, N & Marsland, A 1988 The accuracy of manual diagnosis for cervical zygapophyseal joint pain syndromes. *Medical Journal of Australia*, 148, pp. 233–236.

Jull, G, Kristiansson, E & Dall'Alba, P 2004 Impairment in the cervical flexors: A comparison of whiplash and insidious onset neck pain patients. *Manual Therapy*, 9, pp. 89–94.

Jull, G, Sterling, M, Falla, D et al. 2008a Alternations in cervical muscle function in neck pain. In *Whiplash, headache and neck pain*. Elsevier, Sydney.

Jull, G, Sterling, M, Falla D et al. 2008b Principles of management of cervical disorders. In *Whiplash, headache and neck pain*. Elsevier, Sydney.

Kay, T, Gross, A, Goldsmith, C et al. 2005 Exercises for mechanical neck disorders. *Cochrane Database of Systematic Reviews*, 3, CD004250.

Lam, SL, Cheong, WY & Tan, KP 1991 Air in the cervical annulus: The lucent cleft sign. *Singapore Medical Journal*, 32, pp. 255–257.

Lord, S, Barnsley, L, Wallis, B et al. 1996 Percutaneous radiofrequency neurotomy for chronic cervical zygapophseal joint pain. *New England Journal of Medicine*, 335, pp. 1721–1726.

Macnab, I 1973 The whiplash syndrome. *Clinical Neurosurgery*, 20, pp. 232–241.

MacVicar, J, Borowczyk, J, MacVicar, A et al. 2012 Cervical medial branch radiofrequency neurotomy in New Zealand. *Pain Medicine*, 13, pp. 647–654.

Manchikanti, L, Kaye, A, Boswell, M et al. 2015 A systematic review and best evidence synthesis of effectiveness of therapeutic facet joint interventions in managing chronic spinal pain. *Pain Physician*, 18, pp. E535–E582.

Mendel, T, Wink, C & Zimny, M 1992 Neural elements in human cervical intervertebral discs. *Spine*, 17, pp. 132–135.

Miller, M, Gehweiler, JA, Martinez, S et al. 1978 Significant new observations on cervical spine trauma. *American Journal of Roentgenology*, 130, pp. 659–663.

Milne, N 1993 Comparative anatomy and function of the uncinate processes in humans and other mammals. PhD thesis, Department of Anatomy and Human Biology, University of WA.

Okada, E, Masumoto, M, Fujiwara, H & Toyama, Y 2011 Disc degeneration of cervical spine on MRI in patients with lumbar disc herniation. *European Spine Journal*, 20, pp. 585–591.

Ortongren, T, Hansson, H, Lovsund, P et al. 1996 Membrane leakage in spinal ganglion nerve cells induced by experimental whiplash extension motion: A study in pigs. *Journal of Neurotrauma*, 13, pp. 171–180.

Osti, OL, Vernon-Roberts, B & Fraser, RD 1990 Annulus tears and intervertebral disc degeneration. *Spine*, 15, pp. 62–67.

Otremski, J, Marsh, J, Wilde, B et al. 1989 Soft tissue cervical injuries in motor vehicle accidents. *British Journal of Accident Surgery*, 20, pp. 349–350.

Panjabi, M, Cholewicki, J, Nibu, K et al. 1998 Simulation of whiplash trauma using whole cervical spine specimens. *Spine*, 23, pp. 17–24.

Panjabi, M, Dvorak, J, Duranceau, J et al. 1988 Three-dimensional movement of the upper cervical spine. *Spine*, 13, pp. 726–730.

Panzer, M, Fice, J & Cronin, D 2011 Cervical spine response in frontal crash. *Medical Engineering and Physics*, 33, pp. 1147–1159.

Parke, WW 1978 The vascular relations of the upper cervical vertebrae. *Orthopedic Clinics of North America*, 9, p. 879.

Pearson, A, Ivancic, P & Panjabi, M 2004 Facet joint cinematics and injury mechanism during simulated whiplash. *Spine*, 29, pp. 393–397.

Penning, L 1968 *Functional pathology of the cervical spine.* Excerpta Medica Foundation, Baltimore.

Penning, L 1978 Normal movements of the cervical spine. *American Journal of Roentgenology*, 130, pp. 317–326.

Persson, M, Sorensen, J & Gerdle, B 2016 Chronic whiplash-associated disorders: Responses to nerve blocks of cervical zygapophyseal joints. *Pain Medicine*, 17, pp. 2162–2175.

Pettersson, K, Hildingsson, C, Toolanen, G et al. 1997 Disc pathology after whiplash injury: A prospective MRI and clinical investigation. *Spine*, 22, pp. 283–288.

Pikus, H & Phillips, J 1995 Characteristics of patients successfully treated for cervicogenic headache by surgical decompression of the second cervical nerve root. *Headache*, 35, pp. 621–629.

Quintner, J 1989 A study of upper limb pain and paraesthesiae following neck injury in motor vehicle accidents. *British Journal of Rheumatology*, 28, pp. 528–533.

Reymond, R, Wheeler, P, Perovic, M et al. 1972 The lucent cleft sign of cervical disc injury or disease. *Clinical Radiology*, 23, pp. 188–192.

Schneider, G, Smith, A, Hooper, A et al. 2010 Minimising the source of nociception and its concurrent effect on sensory hypersensitivity: An exploratory study in chronic whiplash patients. *BMC Musculoskeletal Disorders*, 11, p. 29.

Schonstrom, N, Twomey, L & Taylor, J 1993 The lateral atlanto-axial joints and their synovial folds: An in vitro study of soft tissue injuries and fractures. *Journal of Trauma*, 35, pp. 886–892.

Scott, D, Jull, G & Sterling, M 2005 Hypersensitivity is a feature of chronic whiplash associated disorders but not of chronic idiopathic neck pain. *Clinical Journal of Pain*, 21, pp. 175–181.

Scott, J, Boswirth, TR, Cribb, AM et al. 1994 The chemical morphology of age-related changes in human intervertebral disc glycosaminoglycans from cervical, thoracic and lumbar nucleus pulposus and annulus fibrous. *Journal of Anatomy*, 184, pp. 73–82.

Sivola, S, Levoska, O, Tervonen, O et al. 2002 MRI changes of cervical spine in asymptomatic and symptomatic young adults. *European Spine Journal*, 11, pp. 358–363.

Smith, A, Jull, G, Schneider, G et al. 2014 Cervical radiofrequency neurotomy reduces central hyperexcitability and improves neck movement in individuals with chronic whiplash. *Pain Medicine*, 15, pp. 128–141.

Smith, A, Jull, G, Scheider, G et al. 2016 Low pain catastrophization and disability predict successful outcome to radiofrequency neurotomy in individuals with chronic whiplash. *Pain Practice*, 16, pp. 311–319.

Sterling, M 2003 Motor sensory and psychological impairments following whiplash injury. PhD thesis, Department of Physiotherapy, University of Queensland.

Svensson, M, Aldman, B, Bostrom, O et al. 1998 Nerve cell damage in whiplash injuries: Animal experimental studies. *Orthhopade*, 27, pp. 820–826.

Taylor, J 1974 Growth and development of human intervertebral discs. PhD thesis, Faculty of Medicine, University of Edinburgh.

Taylor, J 1993 Neck sprain. *Australian Family Physician*, 22, pp. 1623–1629.

Taylor, J 1996 An unpublished measurement study of cervical mid-disc height on 96 adult specimens from young adults to elderly subjects showing loss of height with increased age.

Taylor, J 2002 The pathology of whiplash: Neck sprain. *British Columbia Medical Journal*, 44, p. 253.

Taylor, J 2003 Cervical facet angles: Their influence on disc fissuring and injuries. Proceedings of Inaugural Scientific Symposium, The Adelaide Centre for Spinal Research, September.

Taylor, J & Kakulas, B 1991 Neck injuries. *The Lancet*, 338, p. 1343.

Taylor, J, Kakulas, B & Margolius, K 1992 Road accidents and neck injuries. *Proceedings of the Australasian Society for Human Biology*, 5, pp. 211–231.

Taylor, J & O'Sullivan, P 2000 Lumbar segmental instability: Pathology, diagnosis and conservative management. In Twomey, L & Taylor, J (eds), *Physical therapy of the low back*, 3rd edn. Churchill Livingstone, New York.

Taylor, JR & Taylor, M 1996 Cervical spine injuries: An autopsy study of 109 blunt injuries. *Journal of Musculoskeletal Pain*, 4, pp. 61–79.

Taylor, J & Twomey, LT 1993 Acute injuries to cervical joints. *Spine*, 18, pp. 1115–1122.

Taylor, J & Twomey, L 1994 Functional and applied anatomy of the cervical spine. In Grant, R (ed.), *Physical therapy of the cervical and thoracic spine*, 2nd edn, pp. 1–26. Churchill Livingstone, New York.

Taylor, J & Twomey, L 2000 The natural history of the lumbar spine. In Twomey, L & Taylor, J (eds), *Physical therapy of the low back*, 3rd edn. Churchill Livingstone, New York.

Taylor, J & Twomey, L 2005 Whiplash injury and neck sprain: A review. *Critical Reviews in Physical and Rehabilitation Medicine*, 17, pp. 285–299.

Taylor, J, Twomey, L & Kakulas, B 1998 Dorsal root ganglion injuries in 109 blunt trauma fatalities. *Injury*, 29, pp. 335–339.

Taylor, J, Twomey, L & Levander, B 2000 Contrasts between cervical and lumbar motion segments. *Critical Reviews in Physical and Rehabilitation Medicine*, 12, pp. 345–371.

Taylor, J, Twomey, L & Taylor, M 1992 Sectioning osteo-ligamentous tissue blocks. Proceedings of the Annual Conference of the Australasian Society for Human Biology, 'Humans on the Move', Australian National University, Canberra.

Taylor, J, Taylor, M & Twomey, L 1996 Letter to the editor. *Spine*, 21, p. 2300.

Tominaga, Y, Ivancic, P & Panjabi, M 2006 Head-turned rear impact causing dynamic intervertebral foramen narrowing: Implications for ganglion and nerve root injury. *Journal of Neurosurgery: Spine*, 4, pp. 380–387.

Tondury, G 1959 La colonne cervicale, son developpement et ses modifications durant la vie. *Acta Orthopaedica Belgica*, 25, pp. 602–626.

Twomey, L & Taylor, J 1984 Old age and physical capacity: Use it or lose it. *Australian Journal of Physiotherapy*, 30, pp. 115–120.

Twomey, L & Taylor, J 1995 Spine care. In White, A & Schofferman, JA (eds), *Spine care*, Vol 2. Mosby, St Louis.

Uhrenholt, L, Grunnet-Nilsson, N & Hartvigsen, J 2002 Cervical spine lesions after road traffic accidents. *Spine*, 27, pp. 1934–1941.

Vanessis, P 1987 *The pathology of neck injuries.* Butterworths, London.

Vernon-Roberts, B, Fazzalari, NL & Manthey, BA 1997 Pathogenesis of tears of the annulus investigated by multiple-level transaxial analysis of the T12–L1 disc. *Spine*, 22, pp. 2641–2646.

Vetti, N, Krakenes, J, Ask, T et al. 2011 Follow-up MR imaging of the alar and transverse ligaments after whiplash injury: A prospective controlled study. *American Journal of Neuroradiology*, 32, 1836–1841.

Wainner, R, Fritz, J, Irrgang, J et al. 2003 Reliability and diagnostic accuracy of clinical examination and patient report measures for cervical radiculopathy. *Spine*, 28, pp. 52–62.

Wallis, B, Lord, S, Barnsley, L et al. 1996 Pain and psychological symptoms of Australian patients with whiplash. *Spine*, 21, pp. 804–810.

Waxman, S & Rizzo, M 1996 The whiplash syndrome: A disorder of dorsal root ganglion neurons? *Journal of Neurotrauma*, 13, pp. 735–739.

Yukuwa, Y, Kato, F, Suda, K et al. 2012 Age-related changes in osseous anatomy, alignment, and range of motion of the cervical spine. Part I: Radiographic data from over 1200 asymptomatic subjects. *European Spine Journal*, 21, pp. 1482–1498.

Zejda, J & Bartolomiej, S 2003 Cervical spine degenerative changes in coal miners. *International Journal of Occupational Medicine and Environmental Health*, 16, pp. 49–53.

INDEX

Page numbers followed by *f* or *t* indicate figures or tables.

whiplash-associated disorder
  (WAD) — *cont.*
  rim lesion in 148–149,
    149–152f, 153, 153f
  vacuum cleft in 151f, 168, 169f
  zygapophyseal facet 'hot spots'
    and 174
women
  disc herniation in 107f
  dorsal root ganglion injury in
    127f
  facet fracture in 139f
  high central cord injury in 124f

multifidus muscle in 140f
rim lesion in 96f
spinal stenosis in 89f
spontaneous interbody fusion
  in 93f

X

x-ray 3, 147–148, 151f, 153, 155,
  159, 168, 174

Y

young adult 95
  C1–2 joint in 20f, 21f

cervical spine in 46–52f, 49
disc height in 82
discography of 80f
facet injury in 112–118f
fissure in 82, 177
herniation in 107f
rim lesion in 96–97f
zygapophyseal facet joint in 53

Z

zygapophyseal facet joint 2, 22f,
  25f, 40f, 53, 90f, 174, 178